A Series of Textbooks for Public Health

EPIDEMIOLOGY

流行病学

赵进顺　倪春辉　王建明　/主编

ZHEJIANG UNIVERSITY PRESS
浙江大学出版社

图书在版编目(CIP)数据

流行病学 = Epidemiology：英文 / 赵进顺，倪春辉，王建明主编. —杭州：浙江大学出版社，2020.7
ISBN 978-7-308-20303-6

Ⅰ.①流… Ⅱ.①赵… ②倪… ③王… Ⅲ.①流行病学－医学院校－教材－英文 Ⅳ.①R18

中国版本图书馆 CIP 数据核字(2020)第 106431 号

流行病学

赵进顺　　倪春辉　　王建明　　主编

丛书策划	朱　玲
责任编辑	郑成业
责任校对	董齐琪　虞雪芬
封面设计	春天书装
出版发行	浙江大学出版社
	（杭州市天目山路 148 号　邮政编码 310007）
	（网址：http://www.zjupress.com）
排　　版	浙江时代出版服务有限公司
印　　刷	杭州钱江彩色印务有限公司
开　　本	787mm×1092mm　1/16
印　　张	15.5
字　　数	490 千
版 印 次	2020 年 7 月第 1 版　2020 年 7 月第 1 次印刷
书　　号	ISBN 978-7-308-20303-6
定　　价	49.00 元

Contributors

叶海亚·阿布卡里亚/Abqariyah，Yahya（马来亚大学医学院社会和预防医学系/Department of Social and Preventive Medicine，Faculty of Medicine，University of Malaya）

艾自胜/Ai，Zisheng（同济大学医学院医学统计学教研室/Department of Medical Statistics，School of Medicine，Tongji University）

柏建岭/Bai，Jianling（南京医科大学公共卫生学院生物统计学系/Department of Biostatistics，School of Public Health，Nanjing Medical University）

珍妮·鲍曼/Bowman，Jenny（自由撰稿人和编者 freelance writer and editor）

岑晗/Cen，Han（宁波大学医学院公共卫生学院/School of Public Health，Medical School of Ningbo University）

戴悦/Dai，Yue（福建医科大学公共卫生学院卫生管理学系/Department of Health Management，Public Health School，Fujian Medical University）

黄民耀/Derry，Minyao Ng（宁波大学医学院/Medical School of Ningbo University）

丁玉松/Ding，Yusong（石河子大学医学院预防医学系/Department of Preventive Medicine，School of Medicine，Shihezi University）.

董长征/Dong，Changzheng（宁波大学医学院公共卫生学院/School of Public Health，Medical School of Ningbo University）

范引光/Fan，Yinguang（安徽医科大学公共卫生学院流行病与卫生统计学系/Department of Epidemiology and Health Statistics，School of Public Health，Anhui Medical University）

冯丹/Feng，Dan（中山大学公共卫生学院营养学系/Department of Nutrition，School of Public Health，Sun Yat-sen University）

冯晴/Feng，Qing（南京医科大学公共卫生学院营养与食品卫生学系/Department of Nutrition and Food Hygiene，School of Public Health，Nanjing Medical University）

凤志慧/Feng，Zhihui（山东大学公共卫生学院职业与环境健康学系/Department of Occupational and Environmental Health，School of Public Health，Shandong University）

郭欣/Guo，Xin（山东大学公共卫生学院卫生毒理与营养学系/Department of Toxicology and Nutrition，School of Public Health，Shandong University）

玛丽亚·哈莱姆/Haleem，Maria（宁波大学医学院/Medical School of Ningbo University）

韩丽媛/Han，Liyuan（中国科学院大学华美医院，中国科学院大学宁波生命与健康产业研究院/Hwa Mei Hospital，Ningbo Institute of Life and Health Industry，University of Chinese Academy of Sciences）

何灿霞/He，Canxia（宁波大学医学院公共卫生学院/School of Public Health，Medical School of Ningbo University）

何斐/He，Fei（福建医科大学公共卫生学院流行病与卫生统计学系/Department of Epidemiology and Health Statistics，Public Health School，Fujian Medical University）

胡付兰/Hu，Fulan（深圳大学医学部公共卫生学院流行病与卫生统计学教研室/Department of Epidemiology and Biostatistics，School of Public Health，Health Science Center，Shenzhen University）

华启航/Hua，Qihang（宁波大学医学院公共卫生学院/School of Public Health，Medical School of Ningbo University）

荆春霞/Jing，Chunxia（暨南大学基础医学院公共卫生与预防医学系/Department of Public Health and Preventive Medicine，School of Medicine，Jinan University）

敬媛媛/Jing，Yuanyuan（川北医学院预防医学系/Department of Preventive Medicine，North Sichuan Medical College）

孔璐/Kong，Lu（东南大学公共卫生学院劳动卫生与环境卫生学系/Department of Occupational and Environmental Health，School of Public Health，Southeast University）

冷瑞雪/Leng，Ruixue（安徽医科大学公共卫生学院流行病与卫生统计学系/Department of Epidemiology and Health Statistics，School of Public Health，Anhui Medical University）

李煌元/Li，Huangyuan（福建医科大学公共卫生学院预防医学系/Department of Preventive Medicine，Public Health School，Fujian Medical University）

李京/Li，Jing（潍坊医学院公共卫生学院预防医学系环境卫生教研室/Division of Environmental Health，Department of Preventive Medicine，School of Public Health，Weifang Medical University）

李静/Li，Jing（徐州医科大学公共卫生学院卫生学系/Department of Hygiene，School of Public Health，Xuzhou Medical University）

李举双/Li，Jushuang（温州医科大学公共卫生与管理学院预防医学系/Department of Preventive Medicine，School of Public Health and Management，Wenzhou Medical University）

李晓枫/Li，Xiaofeng（大连医科大学公共卫生学院流行病学教研室/Department of Epidemiology，School of Public Health，Dalian Medical University）

李永华/Li，Yonghua（济宁医学院公共卫生学院食品安全与健康教研室/Department of Food Safety and Health，School of Public Health，Jining Medical University）

李育平/Li，Yuping（扬州大学临床医学院，江苏省苏北人民医院/Clinical Medical School of Yangzhou University，Northern Jiangsu People's Hospital）

李真/Li，Zhen（宁波大学医学院公共卫生学院/School of Public Health，Medical School of Ningbo University）

廖奇/Liao，Qi（宁波大学医学院公共卫生学院/School of Public Health，Medical School of Ningbo University）

林玉兰/Lin，Yulan（福建医科大学公共卫生学院流行病与卫生统计学系/Department of Epidemiology and Health Statistics，Public Health School，Fujian Medical University）

刘丽亚/Liu，Liya（宁波大学医学院公共卫生学院/School of Public Health，Medical School of Ningbo University）

卢光玉/Lu，Guangyu（扬州大学医学院预防医学系/Department of Preventive Medicine，Medical College of Yangzhou University）

马俊香/Ma，Junxiang（首都医科大学公卫学院劳动卫生与环境卫生学系/Department of Occupational and Environmental Health，School of Public Health，Capital Medical University）

马儒林/Ma，Rulin（石河子大学医学院预防医学系/Department of Preventive Medicine，School of Medicine，Shihezi University）

安妮·马穆沙什维利/Mamuchashvili，Anny（宁波大学医学院/Medical School of Ningbo University）

毛广运/Mao，Guangyun（温州医科大学公共卫生与管理学院预防医学系，温州医科大学附属眼视光医院临床研究中心/Department of Preventive Medicine，School of Public Health and Management，and Center on Clinical Research of the Eye Hospital，Wenzhou Medical University）

毛盈颖/Mao，Yingying（浙江中医药大学公共卫生学院流行病与卫生统计学教研室/Department of Epidemiology and Health Statistics，School of Public Health，Zhejiang Chinese Medical University）

孟琼/Meng，Qiong（昆明医科大学公共卫生学院流行病与卫生统计学系/Department of Epidemiology and Health Statistics，School of Public Health，Kunming Medical University）

孟晓静/Meng，Xiaojing（南方医科大学公共卫生学院职业卫生与职业医学系/Department of Occupational Health and Occupational Medicine，School of Public Health，Southern Medical University）

倪春辉/Ni，Chunhui（南京医科大学公共卫生学院实验教学中心/Experimental Teaching Center，School of Public Health，Nanjing Medical University）

潘红梅/Pan，Hongmei（昆明医科大学公共卫生学院营养与食品科学系/Department of Nutrition and Food Science，School of Public Health，Kunming Medical University）

庞道华/Pang，Daohua（济宁医学院公共卫生学院营养与食品卫生学教研室/Department of Nutrition and Food Hygiene，School of Public Health，Jining Medical University）

培尔顿·米吉提/Peierdun，Mijiti（新疆医科大学公共卫生学院流行病学教研室/Department of Epidemiology，School of Public Health，Xinjiang Medical University）

仇梁林/Qiu，Lianglin（南通大学公共卫生学院营养与食品卫生学系/Department of Nutrition and Food Hygiene，School of Public Health，Nantong University）

曲泉颖/Qu，Quanying（锦州医科大学公共卫生学院流行病学教研室/Department of Epidemiology，School of Public Health，Jinzhou Medical University）

邵方/Shao，Fang（南京医科大学公共卫生学院生物统计学系/Department of Biostatistics，School of Public Health，Nanjing Medical University）

沈冲/Shen，Chong（南京医科大学公共卫生学院流行病学系/Department of Epidemiology，

School of Public Health，Nanjing Medical University）

施红英/Shi，Hongying（温州医科大学公共卫生与管理学院预防医学系/Department of Preventive Medicine，School of Public Health and Management，Wenzhou Medical University）

孙桂菊/Sun，Guiju（东南大学公共卫生学院营养与食品卫生学系/Department of Nutrition and Food Hygiene，School of Public Health，Southeast University）

孙桂香/Sun，Guixiang（徐州医科大学公共卫生学院流行病与卫生统计学系/Department of Epidemiology and Health Statistics，School of Public Health，Xuzhou Medical University）

孙宏鹏/Sun，Hongpeng（苏州大学医学部公共卫生学院少儿卫生与社会医学系/Department of Child Health and Social Medicine，School of Public Health，Medical College of Soochow University）

孙鲜策/Sun，Xiance（大连医科大学公共卫生学院劳动卫生与环境卫生教研室/Department of Occupational and Environmental Health，School of Public Health，Dalian Medical University）

唐春兰/Tang，Chunlan（宁波大学医学院公共卫生学院/School of Public Health，Medical School of Ningbo University）

唐少文/Tang，Shaowen（南京医科大学公共卫生学院流行病学系/Department of Epidemiology，School of Public Health，Nanjing Medical University）

童智敏/Tong，Zhimin（昆山疾病预防控制中心/Kunshan Municipal Center for Disease Control and Prevention）

王春平/Wang，Chunping（潍坊医学院公共卫生学院预防医学系/Department of Preventive Medicine，School of Public Health，Weifang Medical University）

王辉/Wang，Hui（北京大学医学部公共卫生学院妇幼卫生系/Department of Maternal and Children Health，School of Public Health，Peking University Health Science Center）

王建明/Wang，Jianming（南京医科大学公共卫生学院流行病学系/Department of Epidemiology，School of Public Health，Nanjing Medical University）

王津涛/Wang，Jintao（四川大学华西公共卫生学院环境卫生与职业医学系/Department of Environmental Health and Occupational Medicine，West China School of Public Health，Sichuan University）

王乐三/Wang，Lesan（中南大学湘雅公共卫生学院流行病与卫生统计学系/Department of Epidemiology and Health Statistics，Xiangya School of Public Health，Central South University）

王丽君/Wang，Lijun（暨南大学医学院公共卫生与预防医学系/Department of Public Health and Preventive Medicine，School of Medicine，Jinan University）

王强/Wang，Qiang（江苏大学医学院预防医学与卫生检验系/Department of Preventive Medicine and Public Health Laboratory Science，School of Medicine，Jiangsu University）

王少康/Wang，Shaokang（东南大学公共卫生学院营养与食品卫生学系/Department of

Nutrition and Food Hygiene，School of Public Health，Southeast University)

王涛/Wang，Tao（温州医科大学公共卫生与管理学院预防医学系/Department of Preventive Medicine，School of Public Health and Management，Wenzhou Medical University)

王晓珂/Wang，Xiaoke（南通大学公共卫生学院职业医学与环境毒理学系/Department of Occupational Medicine and Environmental Toxicology，School of Public Health，Nantong University)

王子云/Wang，Ziyun（贵州医科大学公共卫生学院流行病与卫生统计学系/Department of Epidemiology and Health Statistics，School of Public Health，Guizhou Medical University)

黄丽冰/Wong，Li Ping（马来亚大学医学院社会和预防医学系/Department of Social and Preventive Medicine，Faculty of Medicine，University of Malaya)

吴冬梅/Wu，Dongmei（南京医科大学公共卫生学院职业医学与环境卫生学系/Department of Occupational Medicine and Environmental Health，School of Public Health，Nanjing Medical University)

吴继国/Wu，Jiguo（南方医科大学公共卫生学院环境卫生学系/Department of Environmental Health，School of Public Health，Southern Medical University)

吴秋云/Wu，Qiuyun（徐州医科大学公共卫生学院卫生学系/Department of Hygiene，School of Public Health，Xuzhou Medical University)

吴思英/Wu，Siying（福建医科大学公共卫生学院流行病与卫生统计学系/Department of Epidemiology and Health Statistics，School of Public Health，Fujian Medical University)

吴莹/Wu，Ying（南方医科大学生物统计教研室/Department of Biostatistics，Southern Medical University)

肖艳杰/Xiao，Yanjie（锦州医科大学公共卫生学院流行病学系/Department of Epidemiology，School of Public Health，Jinzhou Medical University)

徐进/Xu，Jin（宁波大学医学院公共卫生学院/School of Public Health，Medical School of Ningbo University)

许望东/Xu，Wangdong（西南医科大学公共卫生学院循证医学中心/Department of Evidence-Based Medicine，School of Public Health，Southwest Medical University)

严玮文/Yan，Weiwen（南京医科大学公共卫生学院预防医学实验教学中心/Experimental Teaching Center of Preventive Medicine，School of Public Health，Nanjing Medical University)

杨丹婷/Yang，Danting（宁波大学医学院公共卫生学院/School of Public Health，Medical School of Ningbo University)

杨艳/Yang，Yan（西南医科大学公共卫生学院营养与食品卫生教研室/Department of Nutrition and Food Hygiene，School of Public Health，Southwest Medical University)

姚美雪/Yao，Meixue（徐州医科大学公共卫生学院流行病与卫生统计学系/Department of Epidemiology and Health Statistics，School of Public Health，Xuzhou Medical University)

叶洋/Ye，Yang（江苏大学医学院预防医学与卫生检验系/Department of Preventive Medicine and Public Health Laboratory Science，School of Medicine，Jiangsu University）

易洪刚/Yi，Honggang（南京医科大学公共卫生学院生物统计学系/Department of Biostatistics，School of Public Health，Nanjing Medical University）

尹洁云/Yin，Jieyun（苏州大学医学部公共卫生学院流行病与卫生统计学教研室/Department of Epidemiology and Health Statistics，School of Public Health，Medical College of Soochow University）

于广霞/Yu，Guangxia（福建医科大学公共卫生学院预防医学系/Department of Preventive Medicine，School of Public Health，Fujian Medical University）

俞琼/Yu，Qiong，（吉林大学公共卫生学院流行病与卫生统计学教研室/Department of Epidemiology and Health Statistics，School of Public Health，Jilin University）

袁芝琼/Yuan，Zhiqiong（大理大学公共卫生学院营养与食品卫生学教研室/Department of Nutrition and Food Hygiene，School of Public Health，Dali University）

曾芳芳/Zeng，Fangfang（暨南大学医学院公共卫生与预防医学系/Department of Public Health and Preventive Medicine，School of Medicine，Jinan University）

查龙应/Zha，Longying（南方医科大学公共卫生学院营养与食品卫生学系/Department of Nutrition and Food Hygiene，School of Public Health，Southern Medical University）

张丹丹/Zhang，Dandan（浙江大学基础医学院病理学与病理生理学系/Department of Pathology and Pathophysiology，School of Basic Medical Sciences，Zhejiang University）

张俊辉/Zhang，Junhui（西南医科大学公共卫生学院流行病与卫生统计学教研室/Department of Epidemiology and Health Statistics，School of Public Health，Southwest Medical University）

张莉娜/Zhang，Lina（宁波大学医学院公共卫生学院/School of Public Health，Medical School of Ningbo University）

张利平/Zhang，Liping（潍坊医学院公共卫生学院预防医学系环境卫生教研室/Division of Environmental Health，Department of Preventive Medicine，School of Public Health，Weifang Medical University）

张巧/Zhang，Qiao（郑州大学公共卫生学院卫生毒理学教研室/Department of Toxicology，School of Public Health，Zhengzhou University）

张思懋/Zhang，Simin（南京医科大学公共卫生学院社会医学和健康教育系/Department of Social Medicine and Health Education，School of Public Health，Nanjing Medical University）

张晓宏/Zhang，Xiaohong（宁波大学医学院公共卫生学院/School of Public Health，Medical School of Ningbo University）

赵进顺/Zhao，Jinshun（宁波大学医学院公共卫生学院/School of Public Health，Medical School of Ningbo University）

赵苒/Zhao，Ran（厦门大学公共卫生学院预防医学系/Department of Preventive Medicine，School of Public Health，Xiamen University）

赵秀兰/Zhao，Xiulan（山东大学公共卫生学院营养与毒理学系/Department of Nutrition and Toxicology，School of Public Health，Shandong University）

赵研/Zhao，Yan（匹兹堡大学医学中心/University of Pittsburgh Medical Center）

郑馥荔/Zheng，Fuli（福建医科大学公共卫生学院预防医学系/Department of Preventive Medicine，School of Public Health，Fujian Medical University）

仲崇科/Zhong，Chongke（苏州大学医学部公共卫生学院流行病与卫生统计学教研室/Department of Epidemiology and Health Statistics，School of Public Health，Medical College of Soochow University）

周舫/Zhou，Fang（郑州大学公共卫生学院劳动卫生教研室/Department of Occupational Health，School of Public Health，Zhengzhou University）

周志衡/Zhou，Zhiheng（广州市华立科技职业学院健康学院/Health College of Guangzhou Huali Science and Technology Vocational College；深圳市福田区第二人民医院/ The Second People's Hospital of Futian District，Shenzhen）

邹祖全/Zou，Zuquan（宁波大学医学院公共卫生学院/School of Public Health，Medical School of Ningbo University）

Preface

Public health is the science and art of disease prevention. It targets many facets necessary to the well-being of society, including prolonging life, the promotion of physical health through organized community efforts directed at environmental sanitation, the control of community infections, the education of the individual in the principles of personal hygiene, the development of the social machinery to ensure that every individual in the community has an adequate standard of living for the maintenance of health, and the organization of medical and nursing services to aid early diagnosis and enable preventive treatment of diseases. Public health includes many sub-branches, among which the most important ones are preventive medicine, medical statistics, epidemiology, and health services. Preventive medicine is an important part of medical science, which, when integrated with basic medicine and clinical medicine, forms the entire frame of modern medicine. Because preventive medicine, medical statistics, and epidemiology are three important compulsory subjects for international students majoring in clinical medicine, Zhejiang University Press organized public health experts from five universities in China and the University of Texas in the United States of America to compile an English textbook entitled *Preventive Medicine*, *Medical Statistics and Epidemiology*, which was published in 2014. In recent years, this textbook has played an important role in teaching preventive medicine, medical statistics, and epidemiology to international students majoring in clinical medicine in China.

With the continuous expansion and internationalization of higher education in China and many developments in preventive medicine, medical statistics, and epidemiology, a revised edition of this important textbook was required. In 2018, Zhejiang University Press organized experts to reprint the textbook. For the revised edition, the quality was raised significantly to meet global demands. The authors endeavor to improve the quality of this textbook and reflect the latest developments in the fields of preventive medicine, medical statistics, and epidemiology. In addition, the authors present a resource to standardize and unify the quality of teaching and materials for international students majoring in clinical medicine in China.

The new edition is a series of textbooks for public health including *Preventive Medicine*, *Medical Statistics*, and *Epidemiology*.

This book, *Epidemiology*, includes 13 chapters and describes the basic theory of epidemiology, commonly used research methods, disease prevention and control. Chapter 1 introduces the definition, history, and common research methods used in epidemiology, as well as the application and characteristics of epidemiology. Chapter 2 is about the distribution of diseases including measures of disease frequency, patterns of disease distribution and the environmental intensity of diseases. Chapters 3, 4, and 5 systematically introduce three basic epidemiological research methods: descriptive study, cohort study, and case-control study, including the basic principles, designs, quality control, applications, methods of data analysis, strengths, and limitations of each method. Chapter 6 is about experimental studies and introduces the basic principle, design, implementation, and various biases that can exist in clinical trials, as well as the advantages, disadvantages, and possible ethical issues in an experimental study. Chapter 7 introduces the causal influence, including the causal models, information, and criteria. Chapter 8 is about the diagnostic test and includes the definition, design, and evaluation of a diagnostic test. This chapter also briefly discusses the differences between a diagnostic test and a screening test and compares the bias of these two tests. Chapter 9 is about communicable diseases and includes etiology, the infectious process, and spectrum of communicable diseases. This chapter emphasizes the relationship between the epidemic process, prevention, and control of communicable diseases. Chapter 10 is about the various noncommunicable diseases (NCDs), and introduces the various epidemiological characteristics, prevention and control of NCDs. Chapter 11 introduces molecular epidemiology and includes the definition, research content and methods of molecular epidemiology. Chapter 12 focuses on both systematic review and meta-analysis, and introduces the basic knowledge, essential steps, and reporting guidelines of systematic reviews. This chapter also discusses the basic concept and process of meta-analysis, and its advantages and disadvantages. Chapter 13 discusses the interpretation of epidemiologic literature and shows the reader the appropriate method to perform a literature search, review individual studies and establish a causal relationship. Through the study of this book, the reader will learn how to use epidemiological methods to study the occurrence, development, and distribution of diseases in specific populations, and propose measures to control diseases and promote health.

In addition to this textbook, a concise bilingual manual with *pinyin* has been compiled. The authors envision this manual to be useful in bridging the language barrier faced by international students studying clinical medicine in China, especially those starting internships in Chinese hospitals, or by Chinese doctors who intend to practice in a foreign country and wish to have a convenient guide to refer to while practicing. This manual consists of the following parts: Part 1 includes a translation of all laboratory reports used in Chinese hospitals, which are categorized by department for ease of use, how to interpret each report, and the normal values; Part 2 consists of questions to ask during history taking in both English and Chinese with *pinyin*, to allow a doctor or intern to obtain information despite the language barrier; Part 3 includes various tips and checklists of the most common physical examination; Part 4 lists the common communication skills necessary for various patient scenarios, including but not limited to "Breaking Bad News" and "Explaining

Medication"; Part 5 consists of case report forms (discharge summary for hospitalized patients and medical records for outpatient department); Part 6 is a guide on the use of the basic Chinese hospital software; Part 7 shows clinical formulae needed in the clinical practice. This manual will be easy and convenient to use and ensures that any student or doctor have quick and easy access to topics of interest.

In addition, courseware presented in MS PowerPoint is available to supplement this book. And a question bank can be accessed by scanning the QR code at the end of each chapter. Institutions that use this book as teaching material can contact Zhejiang University Press.

More than 40 institutions of higher education both in China and abroad participated in the compilation of this series of textbooks. This series of textbooks is the crystallization of the knowledge and experience of experts in the field of public medicine from countries such as China, the United States of America, and Malaysia. All editorial committees pooled their best efforts together to ensure that this series of textbooks is not only innovative but also practical and reflects the latest developments in the related fields.

Finally, a special thanks goes to Mrs. Linda Bowman for her wonderful help in the process of reviewing the manuscript.

However, due to limited time, mistakes and omissions in the books are inevitable; therefore we sincerely seek the readers' feedback. For comments and suggestions, please email: zhaojinshun@nbu. edu. cn

Zhao Jinshun, Ni Chunhui, Wang Jianming

Contents

Chapter 1　Introduction

Epidemiology is the basic science of public health. It is a highly quantitative discipline based on principles of statistics and scientific research methodologies. Epidemiologists describe the distribution of frequencies and patterns of diseases or health events within groups in a population. They use descriptive epidemiology to characterize diseases or health events in terms of time, place and person. They also use analytical epidemiology to search for causes or factors that are associated with an increased risk or probability of disease. Here, the questions of "who" "what" "where" and "when" go to "how" and "why".

Any good news story, whether it is about an aircraft accident, citizen protest march or academy awards ceremony, must include the five ws: what, who, where, when and why to be complete. This also applies to health events, whether it is an outbreak of measles among a kindergarten or the use of PSA (prostate-specific antigen) to screen for prostate cancer among male adults. The difference is that epidemiologists tend to use synonyms for the five ws: health event (what), person (who), place (where), time (when) and causes (why).

1.1　Definition of Epidemiology

The word epidemiology comes from the Greek word *epi* (on or upon), *demos* (people), and *logos* (the study of). In other words, the word epidemiology has its roots in the study of what befalls a population. There are various definitions of epidemiology. However, the following definition, the study of the distribution and determinants of health-related states or events in specified populations and the application of this study to the control of health problems, captures the underlying principles and public health spirit of epidemiology.

The definition of epidemiology has the following characteristics:

①Findings must relate to a specified population.

②Groups rather than individuals are oriented.

③Conclusions are based on comparisons.

④Probability was emphasized.

⑤Psychological and social conditions of subjects are focused on.

⑥The principles of prevention are adhered to.

To understand epidemiology, consider the following three incidents:

①A nurse noted three cases of hepatitis B of unusual origin in a single month at a county health department when reviewing surveillance data in March 1985. Hepatitis B is transmitted through sexual contact by exposure to infected bodily fluids or spread *via* blood, but these three patients did not seem to have the usual risk factors. All three people received injections at the same hospital. The nurse decided to pursue an investigation whether the three cases were related or occurred by chance.

②The director of the department of viral diseases of Center for Disease Control and Prevention (CDC) received a call from a hospital in Philadelphia, Pennsylvania, US on August 2, 1976 in the morning. The nurse reported two cases with severe respiratory illness, and one was fatal. Both of them attended a convention held between July 21 and 24. By the evening of August 2, additional 71 people who attended the same convention had similar symptoms and signs, including acute fever, chills, headache, malaise, cough, and myalgia. 18 conventioneers died between July 26 and August 2, primarily of pneumonia. An investigation began immediately. This incident is known as the first outbreak of Legionnaires' disease which led to the discovery of the pathogen, *Legionella pneumophila*.

③New Mexico physician notified the state health department on October 30, 1989 of three patients with marked peripheral eosinophilia and severe myalgia. They took oral preparations of L-tryptophan, an over-the-counter (OTC) drug sold as a dietary supplement. The disease was characterized as the eosinophilia-myalgia syndrome. The investigation pointed out that L-tryptophan dietary supplements might cause the disease. A suspected agent was identified and the product was taken off the market. Eventually, the problem was traced to a contaminant in the production process at a single manufacturing facility.

1.2   A Brief History of Epidemiology

Epidemiology is gradually formed and developed in the practice of fighting against human diseases, especially infectious diseases. It is an important methodology in the field of modern medicine. It has also obtained fast development in the research fields, contents and methods, with the changes of disease spectrum and medical models.

1.2.1   The Origin of Epidemiology

Epidemiology is an old discipline. The concepts of epidemiology may be traced back more than 2000 years ago. Here, health problems were considered to have spiritual causes and diseases were considered to be the result of sin. The great advance in health practice took place in Greece during the 3rd—4th century BC. The Greek physician Hippocrates (460 BC—380 BC), the father of medicine, sought a logic to sickness. He was the first person known to have examined the relationship between the occurrence of disease and environmental influences. He believed that sickness of the human body is caused by an imbalance of the four humors (air, fire, water and earth "atoms"). He expressed a modern viewpoint in his essay entitled "On Airs, Waters, and Places". His writing provided not only the descriptions of diseases such as tetanus, typhus, and phthisis (now pulmonary tuberculosis) but also an extraordinarily perceptive approach to the causes of diseases. He suggested that environmental factors and host factors are both critical for influencing the occurrence of diseases.

1.2.2   The Formation Period of Epidemiology

The formation period of epidemiology refers to the 18th to 20th century. The 18th century was characterized by an industrial revolution, which led to overcrowding, poor sanitation and subsequent epidemics of infectious diseases. Also various epidemiological applications evolved during this satge.

James Lind (1716—1794), a British physician, was regarded as the founder of naval hygiene in England. He recommended that fresh citrus fruit and lemon juice included in the diet eventually resulted in the eradication of scurvy from the British Navy. In 1754, he published a paper on scurvy when more British sailors were dying of scurvy during wartime than were killed in battle. In a clinical trial, Lind compared the effects of citrus fruits on patients with scurvy against other five alternative remedies and showed that the fruit was evidently better. Thus, he recommended this dietary practice to the Royal Navy. Scurvy disappeared from the ranks when it was finally adopted in 1795.

William Farr (1807—1883), was a British physician who pioneered the quantitative study of morbidity and mortality, establishing the field of medical statistics. Farr is a major figure in the history of epidemiology. He worked for almost 40 years analyzing statistics on death and disease from England and Wales. He is a forerunner of the modern International Classification of Diseases (ICD).

John Snow (1813—1858), was an English physician known for his studies of cholera. He is the father of contemporary epidemiology. His best-known studies include his investigation of London's Broad Street pump outbreak in 1854, and his experiment on waterborne cholera cases receiving water from two regions of London. Snow's innovative approaches to controlling cholera remain valid and are considered exemplary for epidemiologists throughout the world. He showed the harmful effect of contaminated water and suggested intervention strategies to control the epidemic. His ideas and observations were published in his book *On the Mode of Communication of Cholera*.

Edward Jenner (1749—1823), was an English surgeon and the discoverer of the vaccine for smallpox. Smallpox was widespread as a leading cause of death in the 18th century. Jenner noted that a person who had suffered an attack of cowpox (a relatively harmless disease that could be contracted from cattle) could not become infected with smallpox. On May 14, he inoculated an eight-year-old boy, James Phipps, who had never had smallpox. Phipps became slightly ill over the course of the next nine days but was well on the tenth day. On July 1, Jenner inoculated the boy again. No disease developed and protection was complete. He concluded that cowpox not only protected against smallpox but could be transmitted from one person to another as a deliberate mechanism of protection. In 1798, Jenner published a book entitled *An Inquiry into the Causes and Effects of the Variolae Vaccinae*.

John Graunt (1620—1674), founded the science of demography: the statistical study of human populations. He analyzed the vital statistics of London citizens and wrote a book on those figures that influenced the demographers.

1.2.3 The Development Period of Epidemiology

The development of epidemiology has been accelerating since 1940 and could be divided into the following three stages.

1.2.3.1 First Stage

The methods of etiology research for chronic non-communicable diseases developed from 1940s to 1950s. The first example was the study on smoking and lung cancer by Richard Doll and Bradford Hill. In the 20th century, there was an increased incidence of lung cancer, which was attributed to an increase in automobiles, roads, and factories, but the real cause was not known. As British researchers, Doll and Hill, conducted two epidemiological studies to address this. The first, a case-control study in 1947, compared the smoking habit of lung cancer patients with that of other people without lung cancer. The second, a cohort study in 1951, recorded causes of death among British physicians with smoking habits.

Nevertheless, Framingham Heart Study (longitudinal) in Massachusetts, US, in 1948 produced a landmark report on the predictive power of blood pressure, blood cholesterol level, and cigarette smoking for heart and blood vessel diseases. The term "risk factor" is attributed to the investigators of Framingham, who elaborated many central concepts and practical tools in the identification and prevention of elevated cardiovascular risk.

1.2.3.2 Second Stage

Etiology research and analytic designs developed from 1960s to 1980s. New concepts (confounding, bias, and interaction) emerged. Sackett (1979) summarized 35 kinds of potential bias and Miettien (1985) further divided bias into three categories (selection bias, information bias and confounding bias). Jerome Cornfield, established the first multivariate (logistic regression) model during the study of cardiovascular disease in Framingham. In 1983, Last published the first epidemiological dictionary, *A Dictionary of Epidemiology*. In 1986, Rothman published the textbook, *Modern Epidemiology*.

1.2.3.3 Third Stage

Epidemiology is interdisciplinary and its application has been expanding since 1990s with the advancement of biomedical sciences. In the late 20th century, a number of molecular markers were identified as predictors of a certain disease. Kilbourne (1973) termed the epidemiological study on the relationship between biomarkers and diseases as "molecular epidemiology". It became more formalized with the first book *Molecular Epidemiology: Principles and Practice* by Schulte and Perera. Genome-wide association studies (GWAS) identified genetic factors related to diseases and health conditions.

Studies to examine the relationship between an exposure and molecular pathologic signature of disease increased throughout the 2000s. "Molecular Pathology" and "Epidemiology" were integrated to create a new interdisciplinary field of "Molecular Pathological Epidemiology (MPE)", defined as Epidemiology of Molecular Pathology and Heterogeneity of Disease. Heterogeneity of disease pathogenesis will further contribute to elucidate etiologies of the disease. The concept and model of MPE have become widespread in the 2010s.

In etiology and prevention research, systems-type thinking about multiple levels of causation allows epidemiologists to identify contributors and their interactions to the disease. Systems epidemiology is a way to supplement systems biology, with the goal of reducing disease burden at the individual and population levels. It is defined as an epidemiologic approach to risk identification that includes systems-level (omics) exposure measurements, multiple levels (sociodemographic, clinical, biological, etc.), network analyses of inter-relationships among risk factors, and computational simulation of risk scenarios in parallel to data-driven biostatistics risk modeling.

1. 3　Research Methods of Epidemiology

Epidemiology adopts multiple methods used in medicine, sociology, and philosophy with several subjects. It starts by observing or asking the population, then with a description of the frequency and distribution of a disease or health event. The researcher generates hypotheses of the cause of the disease based on these findings. Subsequently, analytic research examines the hypotheses and experimental research confirms the hypotheses. Mathematical model is then used to predict the disease when the occurrence rule of disease is clearly elucidated.

There are three major research methods of epidemiology: observational method, experimental method, and mathematical method. The first two methods are mostly used. The observational method does not impose any intervention measures upon subjects. In other words, this method only observes the distribution characteristics of diseases, health conditions and health-related factors of subjects. It is divided into two subgroups (descriptive research and analytic research) based on whether establishing controls or not. Therefore, there are four subgroups according to design types, including descriptive epidemiology, analytic epidemiology, experimental epidemiology, and mathematical epidemiology. Descriptive epidemiology describes the distribution of diseases or health conditions which reveals the phenomena and gives clues to etiology. Analytic epidemiology examines or demonstrates the hypotheses generated from descriptive epidemiology. In experimental epidemiology, subjects are given intervention measures. This method effectively controls the research conditions, prospectively observes the effect of the intervention, and finally confirms the correlation between susceptible risk factors and diseases. Each method has advantages and disadvantages.

1.3.1　Descriptive Studies

Observational methods include descriptive epidemiology and analytic epidemiology. The former consists of subtypes, including cross-sectional study, disease surveillance, ecological study, and clinical case analysis. Cross-sectional study surveys and collects information about the illness and factors related to the population within a specific time, and then discusses the relationship between factors and illness. This method emphasizes the simultaneous collection of information about illness and related factors. However, reviewing certain habits or special events in the past may explain the correlation between illness and related factors.

Firstly, it describes the distribution characteristics of a disease or health condition in a population which provides evidence for health policy making and preventive measures formulating. Secondly, it describes or analyzes the correlation between related factors and disease/health condition, establishing a foundation for further etiology research. Thirdly, it evaluates the effectiveness of the preventive measure by comparing the altered prevalence of the disease. Finally, it provides a basis for disease surveillance and other epidemiological studies.

The two methods for selecting subjects in a cross-sectional study are census and sampling survey. Census surveys all individuals to the whole population, whereas sampling survey pays attention to a relatively small sample that is randomly selected from the whole population.

1.3.2　Analytic Studies

Analytic epidemiology is composed of case-control study and cohort study. In case-control study design, subjects are divided into the case group and control group. The case group recruits patients with a specific disease, while the control group recruits people without the same disease as patients or the healthy population. The factors that are significantly associated with the disease can be explored by comparing the difference in the exposure between two groups.

With respect to cohort study, subjects are divided into exposure group and control group. Here, one group of the population has exposure and other group without the exposure. The two groups are followed to compare the occurrence of the outcomes to determine whether there is a causal relationship between exposure and outcome, and then estimate the strength of association.

1.3.3　Experimental Studies

Regarding the experimental method, subjects in the study are randomly assigned to different groups (experimental group or control group). Then, participants in the experimental group receive interventions, while participants in the control group do not. After a follow-up period, the outcomes of the two groups are compared and the effects of the intervention are measured. Experimental epidemiology has several characteristics: subjects in the experimental and control group are sampled from the same source population; there is a control group in the study; subjects are randomly assigned to different groups; intervention is artificially imposed; this method is prospective-based, with a reasonable time sequence of exposure and outcomes, allowing for a casual reference. An experimental study in practice should have some basic principles, including the principles of comparison, randomization, blinding and repeat.

There are three subtypes of experimental design according to research purpose and subjects, namely clinical trial, field trial, and community intervention trial. Clinical trial evaluates the effectiveness of medicine/treatment or adverse drug reactions in different groups of patients. For field trial, study subjects are sampled from the general population without specific diseases. It evaluates the effectiveness of preventive measures in a particular situation. The exposure and outcome in the clinical trial and field trial are collected from individuals. The community intervention trial evaluates the effectiveness of interventions by the community or a group of population, not at the individual level. This method considers the overall community population as the intervention unit.

1.4   Application of Epidemiology

1.4.1   Disease Prevention and Health Promotion

Epidemiology is tasked to prevent onset of diseases when the population is disease free, and control, reduce or eliminate a disease after it has happened. Prevention includes a wide range of activities, known as interventions. There are three categories of prevention: primary, secondary and tertiary. Primary prevention aims to prevent disease or injury before it ever occurs. This is done by preventing exposures to risk factors that cause disease or injury, altering unhealthy or unsafe behaviors, and increasing resistance to disease or injury. Secondary prevention plans to reduce the impact of a disease or injury that has already occurred. This is achieved by detecting and treating disease or injury as soon as possible to halt or slow its progress, encouraging personal strategies to prevent reinjury or recurrence, and implementing programs to return people to their original health and function to prevent long-term problems. Tertiary prevention aims to soften the impact of an ongoing illness or injury that has lasting effects. This can be realized by helping people manage health problems and injuries in order to improve their ability to function, increasing their quality of life and prolonging life expectancy.

The role of epidemiology in disease prevention has been of great concern, but its role in health promotion has gained less attention. The World Health Organization (WHO) defines health promotion as "the process of enabling people to increase control over, and to improve their health". Health promotion is the art and science of helping people discover the synergies between their core passions and optimal health, enhancing their motivation to strive for optimal health, and supporting them in changing their lifestyle to move toward a state of optimal health. The epidemiological research which proves the link between unhealthy behavior (tobacco smoking) and disease (lung cancer), and the subsequent health promotion strategies, can reduce the prevalence of the unhealthy behavior (tobacco smoking) and consequently the incidence of disease (lung cancer) significantly.

1. 4. 2　Disease Surveillance

Surveillance consists of many subtypes, including disease surveillance, biological surveillance, behavior surveillance, and environmental surveillance. Biological surveillance surveys samples from whole blood, serum, plasma, saliva, etc. Behavior surveillance collects data on smoking, alcohol drinking, physical activities, sexual behavior or other behaviors. With respect to environmental surveillance, it should pay attention not only to the natural environment but also to the social environment.

Disease surveillance is at the heart of a public health system. It is used to monitor disease trends over time, detect outbreaks, or enrich our knowledge on risk factors that contribute to disease development. It is useful for describing the current status, giving clues to emergency response, providing evidence for decision-making and intervention assessment. Disease surveillance area is either wide or limited so that it takes a long or short time. It monitors only one or more diseases. The collection of surveillance data must be standardized on a national basis in order to be effective and be made available at local, regional and national levels.

China has been establishing a series of surveillance systems since the 1950s. Surveillance for communicable diseases is the main public health activity in China. In 1959, a system for reporting infectious diseases was established. Behavior and chronic non-communicable disease surveillance systems started to emerge in the 1980s. Disease surveillance systems have been recently integrated into the national public health monitoring system.

1. 4. 3　Research for Causes and Risk Factors

Identifying causes or risk factors is important for disease prevention and control. Some diseases, like measles, have a single cause. However, many diseases have multiple causes, for example, hypertension, diabetes, and cancer. Epidemiology seeks to elucidate the risk factors for disease. Sometimes many related risk factors are found while real causes have not been demonstrated. It is well known that smoking can cause lung cancer, but smoking only contributes partly to the development of lung cancer. Controlling smoking has shown significant effectiveness in preventing lung cancer.

1. 4. 4　Research for the Natural History of the Disease

The natural history of the disease is the course that a disease takes in individuals from its pathological onset until its eventual resolution through complete recovery or death. The natural history of a disease can be divided into subclinical stages, a stage with early symptoms, a stage with apparent manifestation, a stage with symptom remission and a stage of recovery. There are several stages with respect to infection, including incubation period, prodromal period, onset stage, and recovery period. The natural history of the disease has theoretical and practical significance in research. For instance, hepatitis B virus is transmitted from a pregnant woman to a newborn baby and then causes acute or even chronic hepatitis. The natural history of hepatitis B provides evidence for immunizing women of childbearing age to prevent hepatitis B in their offspring.

1.4.5   Evaluating the Effectiveness of Disease Prevention and Control

Evaluating the effectiveness of disease prevention and control is an important application of epidemiology. For example, to assess the role of vaccination for children, experimental epidemiology is used to compare the incidence of specific diseases between vaccinated and controlled groups. Researchers can perform large scale interventions in the community. For instance, adding fluorine in drinking water in order to prevent caries, or to prohibit smoking in public areas so as to reduce the incidence of lung cancer.

1.5   Characteristics of Epidemiology

Throughout history, the definition and mission of epidemiology is to solve health problems at different stages. The scope of epidemiological research is expanding and its research methods have improved in recent years. All these suggest that the characteristics of epidemiology have changed and developed. The main characteristics of epidemiology are as follows:

1.5.1   Population

Epidemiology studies the distribution and determinants of health-related states or events in specified populations. It focuses on the population rather than the individual. However, clinical observations determine decisions about individuals. Epidemiological observations relate primarily to groups of people but they also guide decisions about individuals. Outcomes are essential in relation to a population at risk (healthy or sick), cases with the disease under study.

1.5.2   Comparison

The comparison is the core of research methods of epidemiology. Causes or clues of a disease are found from a comparative investigation or analysis (comparing disease rates in groups with different exposures), for example, the incidence of congenital defects before and after a rubella epidemic or the rate of mesothelioma in people with or without exposure to asbestos. Conversely, ascertainment bias creates missed or false clues.

1.5.3 Probability

Epidemiology studies use the relative frequency (incidence and mortality) rather than absolute number to compare the occurrence of health events between populations. Identifying and understanding the causes of disease is the central aim of the discipline of epidemiology. Any condition which increases the probability that a specified event will occur in a given situation is termed as a causative factor. An association between cigarette smoking and lung cancer has been demonstrated since the early 1950s. It does not mean that smoking absolutely causes lung cancer. Here, the causation is probabilistic and multi-factorial.

1.5.4 Social Psychology

Human health correlates with the internal environment in human body as well as the natural environment and social environment. Theoretical development in social epidemiology is organized around factors that influence health, although health research is organized by disease categories or organ systems. Various social factors are relevant to health domains. Epidemiology addresses health outcomes such as chronic disease, infectious disease, mental health, clinical outcomes or disease prognosis. Exposures of social factors include individual-level measures (poverty, education or social isolation), contextual factors (residential segregation or income inequality), and social policies (policies creating income security or promoting educational access).

1.5.5 Prevention

Epidemiology, a subdiscipline of public health and preventive medicine persists in prevention rather than disease treatment. Preventive medicine consists of measures taken for disease prevention. Disease prevention relies on anticipatory actions that can be categorized as primary, secondary, and tertiary prevention.

(Wang Jianming, Xu Wangdong)

Exercise

Chapter 2　Distribution of Disease

The distribution of disease is based on the frequency of a disease and can be influenced by lifestyles, environmental factors, personal characteristics, and others. The distribution of disease may change over time. One of the major tasks in epidemiologic research is to estimate the frequency and distribution of diseases and other health-related events and to measure disease occurrence in relation to various characteristics such as exposure to environmental, occupational, lifestyle factors, genetic traits or other features. The disease distributions in different populations, different regions and different times are the main contents of the descriptive epidemiology and are the starting point of epidemiological research. Understanding the distribution of disease helps us to generate hypotheses about potential causal or preventive factors and to make public health decisions. In this chapter, we will have a comprehensive description of the distribution of diseases.

2.1　Measures of Disease Frequency

2.1.1　Rate and Ratio

2.1.1.1　Rate

In epidemiology, a rate is a measure of how frequently an event occurs in a defined population over a specified period of time. The numerator of a rate is the number of events of interest occurring during a given time period. The denominator is usually the average population size over the same time period.

$$\text{Rate} = \frac{\text{Number of events occurs}}{\text{Average population during the time period}}$$

A rate should include a measure of time, for example, 19/100,000 per year.

The rate can be presented as a crude, specific or standardized one. A crude rate is presented for an entire population, i. e. the overall incidence or mortality rate calculated for a whole population. A specific rate is presented for a sub-group of a population, i. e. age-specific rate, which is a rate for a specified age group. A standardized rate is applied to compare two or more populations with the effects of differences in age or other confounding variables removed. In practice, the standardized rate is the one that would have been seen in a population with a pre-defined distribution of the factor of concern (e. g. , age).

2.1.1.2　Ratio

A ratio is a relationship between two numbers of the same kind (e. g. , objects, persons, units of whatever identical dimension), usually expressed as "a to b" or "a : b". For instance, someone can look at a group of people, count numbers, and refer to the "ratio of men to women" in the group. Suppose there are forty-six people, seven of whom are men. Then the ratio of men to women is 7 to 39. Notice that, in the expression "the ratio of men to women", "men" came first. This order is very important and must be respected. If the expression had been "the ratio of women to men", then the numbers would be "39 to 7".

For another example, supposing the infant mortality rate in the rural area is 16‰, while the infant mortality rate of the urban area is 4‰, thus the relative ratio is 16‰/4‰ = 4, indicating that the infant mortality rate in the rural area is 4 fold of that in the urban area.

2.1.1.3　Proportion

A proportion is a special type of ratio in which the denominator includes the numerator. A proportion can be expressed as a number between 0 and 1 or as a percentage between 0 and 100%. The proportion should not be used as a rate. All proportions are ratios, but not all ratios are proportions. The formula is:

$$\text{Proportion} = \frac{\text{Number of observations of the component}}{\text{Number of observations of the whole}} \times 100\%$$

2.1.2　The Indices of Disease Occurrence

The most common indices of disease occurrence are incidence rate and prevalence rate. These terms are used to refer to rates that measure the frequency of a disease or a health condition in a population. The aim of this section is to explain what each term means, and how the meaning of each term differs.

2.1.2.1　Incidence Rate

The incidence rate (sometimes called incidence) is a measure of the frequency with which a disease occurs in a population over a period of time. The incidence rate of a given disease is the number of persons who develop the disease (number of incident cases) among subjects at risk of developing the disease in the source population over a defined period of time or age. The general formula for the incidence rate is:

$$\text{Incidence} = \frac{\text{Number of new cases in a specified time period}}{\text{Population at risk in this time period}}$$

The "population at risk" is an important term. It refers to an entire study population who could become new cases.

Incidence proportion (also known as cumulative incidence) is the number of new cases within a specified time period divided by the size of the population at risk observed at the beginning of the study. For example, if a population initially contains 1,000 non-diseased persons and 28 develop a condition over two years of observation, then the incidence proportion is 28 cases per 1,000 persons per two years, i. e. 2.8% every two years.

$$\text{Cumulative incidence} = \frac{\text{Number of new cases within a specified period}}{\text{Population at risk at the beginning of the period}}$$

(1)The Numerator and Denominator

The numerator only includes new cases of the disease that have occurred during the specified period and should exclude cases that have already occurred or diagnosed earlier. This is very important when working with chronic infectious diseases.

The denominator is the population at risk. This means that people included in the denominator should have the possibility to develop the disease during the time period. In practice, we usually use census data for the denominator. The denominator should also represent the population from which the cases in the numerator arose.

Some diseases mainly occur in a certain age and gender, under this situation the specific incidence rate is more applicable. Specific incidence rate refers to the calculated incidence according to disease type, age, gender, occupation, or region, etc.

(2)Application of Incidence Rate

The incidence rate is a commonly used indicator, particularly important for the extremely low mortality and non-fatal disease. The incidence rate is usually used to describe the distribution of disease, explore the risk factors, and put forward the assumptions of disease cause and evaluate the effectiveness of prevention measures.

It should be noted that the accuracy of the incidence rate is affected by many factors (i. e. low diagnostic level). When comparing incidence rates of different populations in different regions, we should consider the different distributions in age and gender with a standardized incidence rate.

2. 1. 2. 2   Attack Rate

In epidemiology, an attack rate is the cumulative incidence of infection in a group of people observed over a period of time during an epidemic. Quantitatively, it is the number of exposed people who develop the disease divided by the total number of exposed people. The term should probably not be described as a rate because its time dimension is uncertain. In epidemiology, a rate requires a defined unit change (in this instance, time) over which the rate applies. For this reason, it is often referred to as an attack ratio. For instance, if 70 participants out of 98 became ill in an outbreak, the attack rate was about 71. 4%. The similarity between attack rate and incidence rate is that the numerator is the number of new cases.

$$\text{Attack rate} = \frac{\text{Number of new cases in a specified time period}}{\text{Exposed population in this time period}}$$

The attack rate is useful for comparing the risk of disease in groups with different exposures. The attack rate can be specified for a given exposure. For example, the attack rate in people who consume a certain food is called a food-specific attack rate. It is calculated by:

$$\text{Food-specific attack rate} = \frac{\text{Number of people who ate a certain food and became ill}}{\text{Total number of people who ate that food}}$$

2. 1. 2. 3   Prevalence Rate

Prevalence rate (sometimes called prevalence) is the proportion of people in a population who have a particular disease or condition at a specified point in time, or over a specified period of time. The numerator includes not only new cases but also old cases (people who remained ill during the specified point or period in time). A case is counted in prevalence until death or recovery occurs. This makes prevalence different from incidence, which includes only new cases in the numerator. The denominator of prevalence rate is the total population. The general formula for calculating the prevalence rate is:

$$\text{Prevalence rate} = \frac{\text{Total number of cases in a specified time period}}{\text{Total number in the defined population}}$$

Prevalence ranges between 0 and 1 and has no units.

For example, a study was performed to explore the prevalence of Systemic Lupus Erythematosus (SLE) in the rural area of Anhui Province of China. A total of 1,253,832 individuals were investigated, among which a total of 471 SLE cases were identified. Thus, the prevalence is $471/1,253,832 = 37.56$ per 100,000 persons.

Period prevalence: In epidemiology, period prevalence is the proportion of the population with a given disease or condition over a specific period of time. It could describe how many people in a population had a cold over the cold season in 2006, for example. It is expressed as a percentage of the population and can be described by the following formula:

$$\text{Period prevalence} = \frac{\text{Number of cases that occurred in a given period}}{\text{Number of people during this period}}$$

Point prevalence: In epidemiology, point prevalence is a measure of the proportion of people in a population who have a disease or condition at a particular time, such as a particular date. It is like a snapshot of the disease in time. It can be used for statistics on the occurrence of chronic diseases. This contrasts with period prevalence which is a measure of the proportion of people in a population who have a disease or condition over a specific period of time (i. e. a season or a year). Point prevalence can be described by the formula:

$$\text{Point prevalence} = \frac{\text{Number of existing cases on a specific date}}{\text{Number of population on this date}}$$

(1) Factors that Influence the Prevalence Rate

The prevalence rate is influenced by many factors, such as incidence rate, disease duration, case immigration, healthy control immigration, diagnostic level, or report level (Figure 2.1). But the main factors are the incidence rate and duration of disease. The interrelationship among the prevalence rate, incidence rate and duration of the disease can be described as follows:

$$\text{Prevalence rate } (P) = \text{incidence rate } (I) \times \text{duration of disease } (D).$$

Thus, we can calculate the average duration of disease based on prevalence rate and incidence rate.

For example, a long-term disease (assuming it has a long duration) that was spread widely in a community in 2002 will have a high prevalence at a given point of 2003, but it might have a low incidence rate during 2003 (i. e. lots of existing cases, but not many new ones in that year). Conversely, a disease that is easily transmitted but has a short duration might spread widely during 2002, is likely to have a low prevalence at any given point in 2003.

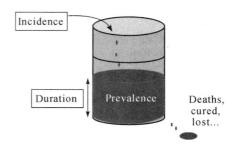

Figure 2.1   The Relationship Between Incidence, Duration and Prevalence

(2) Application of Prevalence Rate

Prevalence estimates are used by epidemiologists, health care providers, government agencies, and insurers. In science, prevalence describes a proportion (typically expressed as a percentage). For example, the prevalence of obesity among American adults in 2012 was estimated by the US Centers for Disease Control (CDC) at approximately 34.9%.

The prevalence rate provides valuable information for the epidemic of chronic diseases with long duration compared to the disease with short duration, which reflects the burden of disease for some populations in a given area (Table 2.1). We can also stipulate the reasonable health facilities and the need for health resources, research the epidemic factors of diseases and evaluate preventive measures of chronic diseases based on prevalence rate.

Table 2.1   Exercise to Fill in the Empty Boxes

Condition	Incidence/100,000 Population/Year	Point Prevalence/ 100,000 Population	Average Duration (Years)
Epilepsy	30		13
Brain tumors	20	65	
Multiple sclerosis		60	12

Which is the commonest (most prevalent) condition?

Which condition has the shortest duration?

(3) Differences Between Prevalence Rate and Incidence Rate

Prevalence is contrasted with incidence, which is a measure of new cases arising in a population over a given period (month, year, etc.). For mnemonic purposes, the difference between prevalence and incidence can be summarized as prevalence answers "How many people have this disease currently?" and incidence answers "How many people per year newly acquire this disease?". The prevalence rate is easier to be obtained than the incidence rate. For example, a population survey can determine how many individuals in a population suffer from a given illness or health condition at a point in time.

Incidence should not be confused with prevalence, which is the proportion of cases in the population at a given time rather than the rate of occurrence of new cases. Thus, incidence conveys information about the risk of contracting the disease, whereas prevalence indicates how widespread the disease is. Prevalence is the proportion of the total number of cases to the total population and is a measure of the burden of diseases on society with no regard to the time at risk or when subjects may have been exposed to a possible risk factor. Prevalence can also be measured with respect to a specific subgroup of a population. Incidence is usually more useful than the prevalence in understanding the disease etiology. For example, if the incidence rate of a disease increases, there is a risk factor that promotes the incidence.

2.1.3　The Indices of Death

2.1.3.1　Mortality Rate

(1) Mortality Rate

The mortality rate is a measure of the number of deaths (in general, or due to a specific cause) in a population, scaled to the size of that population, per unit of time. The mortality rate is typically expressed in units of deaths per 1,000 individuals per year. Thus, a mortality rate of 9.5 (out of 1,000) in a population of 1,000 would mean 9.5 deaths per year in that entire population or 0.95% out of the total. It is distinct from morbidity rate, which refers to the number of individuals in poor health during a given time period (the prevalence rate) or the number of newly appearing cases of the disease per unit of time (incidence rate).

Mortality is the most commonly used indicators for measuring the population death risk. The numerator is the death toll and the denominator is the annual average population. Familiarity with the use and interpretation of mortality rates is necessary.

(2)Crude Mortality Rate

The crude mortality rate (death rate) is the total number of deaths per year per 1,000 people. The crude mortality rate for a given year can be defined as:

$$\text{Crude mortality rate} = \frac{\text{All deaths during the year}}{\text{Population at the mid-year}}$$

For example, in the US in 2003, a total of 2,419,921 deaths occurred. The estimated population was 290,809,777. Then the crude mortality rate in USA in 2003 was 2,419,921/290,809,777, or 832.1 deaths per 100,000 population.

Table 2.2 is an exercise on mortality rate. Region A has much better economic and medical conditions than Region B. Please fill in the empty boxes and answer the following questions. The crude death rates are very similar. Is this the answer you expected? Does this mean, from your perspective, that the risk of death in these two populations are about the same? If your answer to the above question is "No", what reasons can you think of for the similarity in the crude rates?

Table 2. 2   Exercise to Fill in the Empty Boxes

Region	Total Deaths	Mid-Year Population	Death Rate per 1000 Population per Year
A	530,373	52,084,000	
B	3625	345,935	

(3) Category-Specific Mortality Rate

The calculation of mortality rate according to the type of disease, age, gender, occupation and race classification is called category-specific mortality rate. When calculating the category-specific mortality rate, the numerator and denominator must be the corresponding number of populations. When calculating the category-specific mortality rate of myocardial infarction of men over the age of 40, the denominator should be the men over 40 in this area.

The age-specific mortality rate refers to the total number of deaths per year per 1,000 people of a given age. The numerator is the number of deaths in that age group, and the denominator the number of persons in that age group in the population. An age-specific mortality rate is simply the mortality rate for a particular age group. For example, the rate per 1,000 for persons aged 55—65 would be:

$$\frac{\text{Number of deaths in people aged } 55-65}{\text{Mid-year number of people aged } 55-65}$$

(4) Application

Mortality rates have many uses but are often utilized to describe the increase or decrease in a cause of death over a lengthy time period. For instance, the CDC used mortality rates to show that the mortality rate for car-accident deaths in the US dropped from almost 25 per 100,000 to nearly 15 per 100,000 between 1979—2006, while during the same period poisoning deaths rose from 5 to 15 per 100,000. Looking at the mortality rates over time can help health officials understand where to focus on prevention and safety efforts and indicate possible trends in death due to factors affecting the measured population.

The mortality rate of infants and children is often used as a factor to determine the health status of a country. A high infant mortality rate indicates poor prenatal and obstetric care and is often found to be associated with developing nations or regions. In the US, infant mortality rates are often broken down by ethnicity or economic status, to highlight areas where better care is required.

A mortality rate may be used to explain the likelihood of survival or death. This information can help patients decide what treatment will give them the best chance of survival.

A mortality rate may also be expressed as a mortality table, also called a life table. Using a generalized table broken down by age, a mortality table shows the mortality rate and probability of death each year. By looking at a life table, a healthy person can determine the likelihood of death before their next birthday. Life tables are highly generalized and do not include individual factors that may increase or decrease chances of death, such as whether the person smokes, where they live, and if they have a healthy diet or pre-existing medical conditions. At best, mortality tables should be looked at as a rough average of likely lifespan.

The crude mortality rate reflects the total death of a population and is a comprehensive reflection of culture and health level of a region and country. The category-specific mortality rate is a very important indicator in epidemiology, and it is usually used to explore the causes of a disease and evaluate the prevention measures.

2. 1. 3. 2   Fatality Rate

Fatality rate refers to the proportion of patients who die from that illness. It is a measure of the severity of the illness. In epidemiology, a case fatality risk (CFR) is conventionally expressed as a percentage and represents a measure of risk. CFR is most often used for diseases with discrete and limited time courses, such as outbreaks of acute infections. The formula is:

$$\text{Fatality rate} = \frac{\text{Number of cause-specific deaths among the incident cases}}{\text{Number of incident cases}}$$

For instance, under the assumption that 9 deaths occur among 100 people in a community that were diagnosed with the same disease, the CFR, therefore, would be 9%. However, if some of the cases have not yet resolved (either died or recovered) at the time of analysis, this could lead to bias in estimating the CFR.

Technically, CFR is not the rate or ratio and takes values between 0 and 1. If one wants to be very precise, the term "case fatality rate" is incorrect, because the time from disease onset to death is not considered. Nevertheless, the term case fatality rate (and the abbreviation "CFR") is often used in the scientific literature.

In different situations, the denominator of fatality is different. When we calculate disease fatality in hospitalized patients, the denominator is the number of patients discharged from the hospital. While we calculate the fatality of acute infectious disease, the corresponding denominator is the number of patients at the onset of the disease epidemic.

2. 1. 3. 3   Survival Rate

The survival rate is a part of survival analysis, indicating the percentage of people in a study or treatment group who are alive for a given period of time after diagnosis. The survival rate is a proportion of patients in a group who are still alive in a specified period after diagnosis (and is equal to 1—fatality). The survival time is defined as the time that elapsed between diagnosis and death. Survival rates are important for prognosis. Because this rate is based on the population, an individual prognosis may be different depending on newer treatments since the last statistical analysis as well as the overall general health of the patient.

The survival rate is defined as the percent of people who survive a disease such as cancer for a specified amount of time. For example, if the 5-year survival rate for a particular cancer is 34%, this means that 34 out of 100 people initially diagnosed with that cancer would be alive after 5 years. Survival rate does not indicate if cancer is cured or if treatment is completed.

Patients with a certain disease can die directly from that disease or from an unrelated cause such as a car accident. When the precise cause of death is not specified, this is called the overall survival rate or observed survival rate. Doctors often use mean overall survival rates to estimate the patient's prognosis. This is often expressed over standard time periods (i. e. one, five or ten years). For example, prostate cancer has a much higher one-year overall survival rate than pancreatic cancer and thus has a better prognosis.

Note that survival rates are based on statistics and look at the population as a whole. Your prognosis may be different based on many variables such as your general health, and new treatments that have become available. By the time these rates are published, the statistics are frequently several years old.

Estimation of survival depends upon follow-up of diagnosed patients for deaths or withdrawal from observation. There are two related approaches to estimate survival rate: Kaplan-Meier method and Actuarial (life-table) method. In order to fully use the available information through follow-up, survival analysis is mainly used to measure the outcome of various diseases in cohort studies in recent years and to explore the cause of disease with the aid of the life table.

Table 2.3 shows the all-cause and unintentional injury mortality and estimated population by age group, for both sexes and for males alone in the US 2002. Please calculate the following frequency: unintentional-injury-specific mortality rate for both sex; all-cause mortality rate for 25 to 34 years old; all-cause mortality among males; unintentional-injury-specific mortality among 25 to 34 years old males.

Table 2.3　All-Cause and Unintentional Injury Mortality and Estimated Population by Age Group, for Both Sexes and for Males Alone in the US 2002

Age Group (Years)	All Races, Both Sexes			All Races, Males		
	All Causes	Unintentional Injuries	Estimated Pop. (×1000)	All Causes	Unintentional Injuries	Estimated Pop. (×1000)
0—4	32,892	2,587	19,597	18,523	1,577	10,020
5—14	7,150	2,718	41,037	4,198	1,713	21,013
15—24	33,046	15,412	40,590	24,416	11,438	20,821
25—34	41,355	12,569	39,928	28,736	9,635	20,203
35—44	91,140	16,710	44,917	57,593	12,012	22,367
45—54	172,385	14,675	40,084	107,722	10,492	19,676
55—64	253,342	8,345	26,602	151,363	5,781	12,784
65+	1,811,720	33,641	35,602	806,431	16,535	14,772
Not Stated	357	85	0	282	74	0
Total	2,443,387	106,742	288,357	1,199,264	69,257	141,656

Data Source: Web-Based Injury Statistics Query and Reporting System (WISQARS) [online database] Atlanta: National Center for Injury Prevention and Control.

2. 2　Patterns of Disease Distribution

The incidence rate or the epidemic intensity of disease varies in different populations, different regions and different times, due to the influence of pathogenic factors, population characteristics, natural and social environment factors. Some characteristics (gender, ethnicity, etc.) are inherent, while the others are changing with time. The morbidity rate, mortality rate, and fatality rate are associated with the changes of the above characteristics. Distribution characteristics of the disease in different populations are helpful to identify high-risk populations and explore the etiology and epidemic factors of disease.

Compiling and analyzing disease frequency by time, place and person is desirable for several reasons:

①To learn the extent and pattern of the public health problem being investigated and explore which neighborhoods, which months, and which groups of people have the most and least cases.

② To create a detailed description of health status of a population that can be easily communicated with tables, graphs, and maps.

③ To identify areas or groups within the population that have high rates of disease. This information, in turn, provides important clues to the causes of the disease, and these clues can be turned into testable hypotheses.

2. 2. 1　Person

2. 2. 1. 1　Age

Age is a key characteristic in relation to the disease. Both the incidence rate and mortality rate are associated with age.

Populations of different ages are susceptible to different diseases. Children are not only susceptible to respiratory diseases (measles, whooping cough, mumps, etc.) but also susceptible to a large number of recessive infectious diseases (epidemic cerebrospinal meningitis, epidemic encephalitis, and etc.).

The incidence rate of chronic diseases (e. g. , malignant tumor, hypertension, diabetes, and coronary heart disease) increases with age rapidly. There are also age differences about the prevalence of damage. Children and the elderly are prone to drowning and fall injury due to poor reaction ability and young adults are prone to traffic accidents.

When we compare the morbidity rate or mortality rate among different populations, we need to consider the differences of age and use the age-specific rate or standardized rate to avoid bias.

(1) The Purpose of Describing the Age Distribution of Disease

①To identify high-risk populations.

②To explore the epidemic factors and provide clues for disease exploration.

③To analyze the dynamic distribution of age and the immune status of the population.

④To develop prevention measures and evaluate their effects.

（2）Factors accounting for the difference in disease frequency among different age groups

①Susceptibility.

②Opportunity for exposure.

③Latency or incubation period of the disease.

④Physiologic response.

（3）The Methods of Describing the Age Distribution of Disease

Cross-sectional analysis: Cross-sectional analysis (also known as cross-sectional analyses, transversal studies) forms a class of research methods that involve observation of all population, or a representative subset, at one specific point in time. Cross-sectional studies are descriptive ones (neither longitudinal nor experimental).

Cross-sectional studies involve data collected at a defined time. They are often used to assess the prevalence of acute or chronic conditions or to answer questions about the causes of disease or the results of medical intervention. They may also be described as censuses. Cross-sectional studies may involve special data collection, including questions about the past, but they often rely on data originally collected for other purposes. They are moderately expensive and are not suitable for the study of rare diseases. Difficulty in recalling increases information bias.

Cohort analysis: Cohort analysis is a study that focuses on the activities of a particular cohort. If we want to calculate the average income of students over the course of a five-year period following their graduation, we will be conducting a cohort analysis. Cohort analysis allows us to identify relationships between the characteristics of a population and behaviors.

To measure the incidence of disease, we need to start with a group (or cohort) of people who are currently free of the disease of interest but "at risk" of developing it. We then follow them to observe who develop the disease (a cohort study). This analysis is often used in the age distribution of chronic diseases, which especially has great significance in evaluating long-term trends of age distribution. It clearly shows the relationship between pathogenic factors and age, and is helpful in elucidating the effect of age and exposure experience in the frequency of disease.

2.2.1.2　Gender

When we describe the gender distribution of disease, we usually compare the morbidity or mortality rate between men and women. The gender differences in the incidence rate of infectious diseases are mainly caused by different exposure opportunities. For example, the incidence rate of forest encephalitis or epidemic hemorrhage is higher in men compared with women.

The prevalence rate of noncommunicable diseases such as stroke, coronary heart disease and hypertension is higher in men, while cholecystitis and gall-stone are more common in women. The incidence rate of most cancers is higher in men compared to women, except breast cancer, cervical cancer and ovarian cancer. In addition to suicide, the incidence rate of injury is higher in men. The gender difference may be related to different inherent factors (e. g. , genetic, hormonal, anatomic and etc.) or different opportunities or levels of exposure.

2. 2. 1. 3   Occupation

Concerning the relationships between occupation and disease, we may first consider the exposure risk. The economic status and health condition of people with relevant occupation should not be neglected. For example, coal miners are susceptible to silicosis, coking workers are predisposed to lung cancer, herders are susceptible to undulant disease and anthrax, and white-collar workers are predisposed to high blood pressure and coronary heart diseases.

2. 2. 1. 4   Ethnicity

Different ethnicities vary in different aspects, such as genetic, geography, religion, culture, customs and so on. The disease could be affected by these factors. For instance, there are three ethnicities in Malaysia. Lymphoma is more common in Malays, oral cancer is more common in Indians, while nasopharyngeal carcinoma is more common in Chinese.

2. 2. 1. 5   Social Stratification

The occurrence of diseases is related to social factors, which is difficult to quantify. It is made up of many variables such as occupation, family income, educational achievement or census tract, living conditions, and social standing. For example, cerebral embolism often occurs in the wealthy population with a higher economic and cultural level, the incidence rate of stroke is higher among heavy manual labor, and the disability is higher in elderly with low educational level.

2. 2. 1. 6   Marriage and Family

Many previous studies have demonstrated that marital status has an obvious influence on people's health. The incidence rate of cardiovascular disease, suicide and mental disease is higher in divorced populations, demonstrating that divorce has a great influence on people's life.

Family members live together and contact closely. Some infectious diseases (tuberculosis, viral hepatitis, and bacillary dysentery, etc.) are easy to spread in the family. The number of family members, age, gender, immune status, culture background, health level, customs and habits can affect the incidence rate of diseases in a family.

2. 2. 1. 7   Behavior

Unhealthy behaviors, such as tobacco smoking, excessive drinking and drug use, are associated with the risk of diseases. Smoking is a most important factor for lung cancer. The mortality rate of the cancer of throat, pharynx, esophagus, liver, pancreas, or bladder is higher in smokers than non-smokers with a dose-response relationship.

Long-term excessive alcohol drinking has great harm to people's health, especially for liver cirrhosis, esophageal cancer, nasopharyngeal carcinoma, hepatitis, and hypertension. The bone mineral density of alcoholic is reduced, and the risk of hip fracture is $4-8$ times higher than the non-drinkers. Excessive drinking is not only a risk factor for diseases but also an important risk factor for traffic accidents.

2.2.2   Place

The occurring of the disease is often influenced by the natural environment and social living conditions. There are regional differences among the occurrence of various diseases. The distribution characteristics of the disease in different areas reflect the differences in pathogenic factors. Thus, describing the regional difference of a disease may be helpful in providing clues for causes of disease and developing countermeasures.

When we study the regional distribution of a disease, we can define a region according to an administrative division. The unit can be a state, province, municipality, autonomous region, county or town within a country. It is easy to get complete information according to the administrative division. But the adjacent administrative areas may have a similar natural environment, while in the same administrative area the natural environment is different. The region can also be divided according to the natural environment characteristics, such as mountains, plains, lakes, rivers, forests and grassland, etc.

Factors accounting for the geographic variations of disease frequency including natural environment (e. g. , temperature, humidity, rainfall, vegetation, atmospheric pressure, sunshine, and ultraviolet radiation, etc.) or social environment (e. g. , living and working condition, dietary pattern, and healthcare system, etc.).

We can choose the statistical graphs and tables based on the specific situation. When we compare the incidence rate, prevalence rate or mortality rate in different regions, we must consider the standardized rate. At the same time, we should pay attention to the consistency of medical levels, disease registration systems, and diagnostic criteria.

2.2.2.1   Distribution of Disease Between Countries and Within Countries

The distribution of disease is different all over the world. For example, liver cancer is more common in Asia, while the prevalence rate of diabetes is higher in developed countries.

The distribution of disease is also different within a country. For example, the prevalence rate of hypertension is higher in the north than that in the south of China.

2.2.2.2   The Urban and Rural Distribution of the Disease

Many diseases show an obvious difference between urban and rural areas in regional distribution. Because of the convenient traffic and crowded population, respiratory infectious diseases are often popular in cities. For example, in China, most severe acute respiratory syndrome (SARS) cases were mainly concentrated in urban areas. However, the current water supply and sanitation of rural countries are inferior to cities, and the incidence rate of intestinal infectious diseases are significantly higher in rural areas.

2. 2. 2. 3   Endemic

Endemic is the ecological state of being unique to a defined geographic location, such as an island, nation, county or other defined zone. For example, malaria is endemic in tropical regions. The extreme opposite of endemic is cosmopolitan distribution. In epidemiology, an infection is said to be endemic in a population when that infection is maintained in the population without the need for external inputs. Endemic has three types: ① Local endemic. Due to the living habits, health conditions or religions, and etc., the incidence rate of some diseases in some regions is significantly higher than that of other regions for a long time, this kind of situation has nothing to do with the region's natural conditions, and therefore it is called as local endemic. ② Natural endemic, such as skeletal fluorosis and endemic goiter. Due to the influence of the natural environment, certain diseases only exist in certain areas, and this is called natural endemic. ③ Natural foci. The pathogens of disease with natural foci grow well without relying on people.

In order to investigate whether a disease is associated with the local environment, the following points should be noted:

①The incidence rate of the disease is higher in all kinds of people in this area and increases with age.

②The incidence rate of disease is lower in a similar population living in other areas.

③Healthy people after immigrating to this area and living for a period will be affected by this disease and the incidence rate is similar to local residents.

④The incidence rate of the disease will decline when people have emigrated from this area after a certain period.

2. 2. 3   Time

The occurrence of disease changes over time. Some of these changes occur regularly, while others are unpredictable. We can understand the epidemic dynamics of disease through analyzing the time change of disease, and this is helpful to verify the relationship between diseases and possible pathogenic factors. Time distribution of disease can be divided into the following four types.

Rapid fluctuation: The meaning of rapid fluctuation is similar to an outbreak. Outbreak often refers to a smaller range, such as food poisoning in collective canteens, while rapid fluctuation may refer to a wider range. Figure 2. 2 shows a rapid fluctuation of cerebrospinal meningitis in Baoding in 1960s.

Seasonal variation: The frequency of the disease, in relation to or occurring at a certain season or certain seasons of the year, is known as seasonal variation. The incidence rate of disease with seasonal variation is rising in a certain month, such as the incidence rate of respiratory infectious diseases is higher in spring and winter, the incidence rate of intestinal

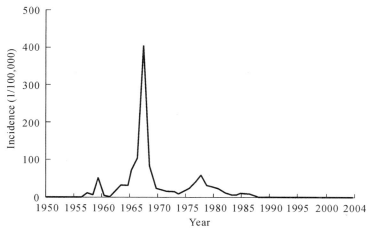

Figure 2. 2   The Incidence of Epidemic Cerebrospinal Meningitis in Baoding (1950—2004)

infectious disease is higher in summer and fall. Some noncommunicable diseases also have seasonal variations (Figure 2. 3). The incidence and mortality rate of stroke is lower in summer and higher in winter. The hemorrhagic cerebral apoplexy is correlated with average temperature negatively, and average pressure positively. The factors that influence the seasonal variation are complicated, including local meteorological factor, lifestyle, health and medical level, etc.

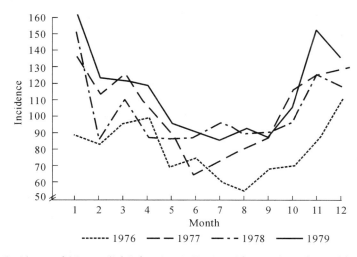

Figure 2. 3   Incidence of Myocardial Infarction in Beijing (the number of monthly distributions)

Periodicity: Periodicity is the tendency to happen or recur at regular intervals. Most infectious respiratory diseases are periodic before the application of effective vaccination. For example, before the large application of the measles vaccine, measles was popular each year in large and medium-sized cities in China.

Secular trend: Secular trend is a concept that refers to a movement or trend in a series over very long periods of time, also known as a long-time trend. Whether something is perceived as a secular variation depends on the available timescale. A secular variation over a time scale of centuries may be part of a periodic variation over a time scale of millions of years (Figure 2. 4). Natural quantities often have both periodic and secular variations. Secular variation is sometimes called a secular trend or secular drift when the emphasis is on a linear long-term trend. Research on the secular trend is helpful in exploring the pathogenic factors of the disease and providing the theoretical basis for disease prevention. Health personnel uses these graphs to assess the prevailing direction of disease occurrence (increasing, decreasing, or essentially flat), evaluate programs, make policy decisions and infer causes of the disease.

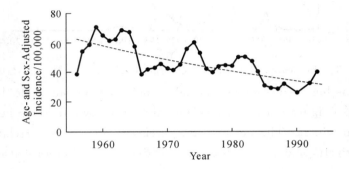

Figure 2. 4   Annual Incidence of Rheumatoid Arthritis in Rochester, MN, US

2. 3   The Epidemic Intensity of Disease

2. 3. 1   Sporadic

Sporadic means occurring at irregular intervals, haphazardly, having no pattern or order in time, appearing in scattered or isolated instances, as a disease. The incidence rate of disease with sporadic is strongly influenced by accidental factors, and the annual incidence rate of these diseases is not stable.

The reasons for sporadic include: ①the disease is popular in this area or residents who have immunity with vaccination; ②the latent infection is dominant; ③the infectious disease has a long incubation period.

2. 3. 2   Outbreak

Outbreak refers to an epidemic limited to a localized increase in the incidence of a disease, e. g. , in a village, town, or closed institution; upsurge is sometimes used as a euphemism for the outbreak.

Outbreak is a term used in epidemiology to describe an occurrence of disease greater than would otherwise be expected at a particular time and place. It may affect a small and localized group or impact upon thousands of people across an entire continent. Two linked cases of a rare infectious disease may be sufficient to constitute an outbreak. Outbreaks may also refer to epidemics, which affect a region in a country or a group of countries, or pandemics, which describe global disease outbreaks.

When investigating disease outbreaks, the epidemiologist has to develop a number of widely accepted steps: verify the diagnosis related to the outbreak; identify the existence of the outbreak (is the group of ill persons normal for the time of year, geographic area, etc.); create a case definition to define who/what is included as a case; map the spread of the outbreak using information technology; develop a hypothesis (what appears to be causing the outbreak?); study the hypothesis (collect data and perform analysis); refine the hypothesis and carry out further studies; develop and implement control and prevention systems; release findings to greater communities.

2.3.3   Epidemic

Epidemic is a widespread outbreak of an infectious disease and many people are infected at the same time. In epidemiology, an epidemic meaning "upon or above" occurs when new cases of a certain disease, in a given human population, and during a given period, substantially exceed what is expected based on recent experience. Epidemiologists often consider the term outbreak to be synonymous with the term epidemic, but the general public typically perceives outbreaks to be more local and less serious than epidemics.

Epidemics of infectious disease are generally caused by a change in the ecology of the host population (e. g. , increased stress or increase in the density of a vector species), a genetic change in the parasite population or the introduction of a new parasite to a host population (by the movement of parasites or hosts). Generally, an epidemic occurs when host immunity to a parasite population is suddenly reduced below that found in the endemic equilibrium and the transmission threshold is exceeded.

An epidemic may be restricted to one location. If it spreads to other countries or continents and affects a substantial number of people, it may be termed as pandemic. The declaration of an epidemic usually requires a good understanding of a baseline rate of incidence. Epidemics for certain diseases, such as influenza, are defined as reaching some defined increase in incidence above this baseline. A few cases of a very rare disease may be classified as an epidemic, while many cases of a common disease (such as the common cold) would not.

(Han Liyuan, Zhong Chongke)

Exercise

Chapter 3　　Descriptive Study

Descriptive studies describe patterns of disease occurrence in relation to variables such as person, place, and time. Descriptive study is a basic to investigate the relationship between cause and effect. Descriptive study systemically describes phenomena to reveal patterns and connections that might otherwise go unnoticed.

3.1　Definition of Descriptive Study

Descriptive study (descriptive epidemiology) is to organize and analyze existing data or some survey data, including the data from experiment, describe the variations in different places, different time and different population character and depict the frequency of disease and health. The data provided by descriptive studies are for public health administrators as well as epidemiologists. Specifically, for public health administrators, knowledge of the populations or subgroups that are most or least affected by disease allows for more efficient allocation of resources and targeting of particular segments of the population for educational and/or prevention programs. For epidemiologists, identification of descriptive characteristics frequently constitutes the important first step in the research for risk factors that can be altered or eliminated to prevent diseases.

Descriptive studies frequently use available information from such diverse sources as census data, vital statistical records, employee health examinations, clinical records from hospitals or private practices, as well as national figures on consumption of foods, medications, or other products. The descriptive studies are normative, correlative, and non-intervention case studies and qualitative studies.

Descriptive studies include ecological study, cross-sectional study, case report and case survey, outbreak survey and screening, etc. However, such studies are limited in their usefulness since no inferences can be made concerning causality. Generally, descriptive epidemiological studies are sentinel devices used to generate hypotheses or to provide evidence that indicates whether there are enough causes for conducting a lengthier and costlier analytic study.

3.2　Cross-Sectional Study

A cross-sectional study examines relationships between diseases (or other health-related conditions) and other variables of interest as they exist in a population at a particular time

(Figure 3. 1). The presence or absence of disease suspected etiologic factors are determined in each member of the study population or in a representative sample at one particular time. Cross-sectional studies are sometimes referred to as "prevalence studies", since they collect data on existing (prevalent) cases of diseases and current characteristics (risk factors) in a population with a certain period of time.

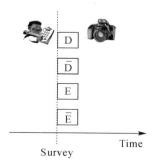

Figure 3. 1   The cross-sectional study is implemented just like a snapshot
in a defined population at a particular point of time.

3. 2. 1   Cross-Sectional Study Methods

Figure 3. 2 is a diagram of the route to design a cross-sectional study.

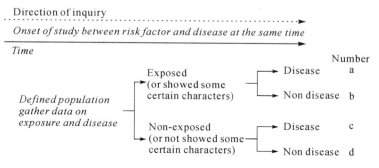

Figure 3. 2   The Route to Design a Cross-Sectional Study

Advantages of cross-sectional study include: used to prove and/or disprove assumptions; not costly to perform and does not require a lot of time; captures a specific point in time; contains multiple variables at the time of the data snapshot; the data can be used for various types of research; many findings and outcomes can be analyzed to create new theories/studies or in-depth research.

Disadvantages of cross-sectional study include: cannot be used to analyze behaviors over a period of time; does not help determine cause and effect; the timing of the snapshot is not guaranteed to be representative; findings can be flawed or skewed if there is a conflict of interest with the funding source; may face some challenges putting together the sampling pool based on the variables of the population being studied.

3. 2. 2　The Purposes and Application of Cross-Sectional Study

The purposes and application of cross-sectional study are as follows:

①To describe the distribution of health conditions and risk factors in different populations and times, thus providing data to guide prevention and control programs.

②To evaluate the associations between risk factors and diseases that can lead to new epidemiologic hypotheses for analytic studies.

③To formulate and evaluate the efforts for public health. For example, data on the distribution of disease might provide important guidance for determining hospital numbers, establishing specialized hospitals, configuring hospital beds, purchasing medical equipment, and determining stockpiles of drugs.

④To provide baseline data that can serve as a basis for subsequent longitudinal studies. Many successful cohort studies grew out from an initial cross-sectional study and then provided more valuable scientific evidence than a single cross-sectional study.

⑤To conduct surveillance. For examples, the health status of a population should be monitored in order to detect cholera cases such as by age, sex, location, water source, and duration of stay in a camp.

⑥To evaluate the health level of a country or an area. For describing rates of injury among children and youth in some area, identifying subgroups of the study population who are at high risk for injury, patterns of childhood injury would be identified consequently, which may be suited to the development and targeting of prevention programs.

3. 2. 3　Design of Cross-Sectional Study

3. 2. 3. 1　To Define the Study Objectives

To define the study objectives is the most important step since it would guide the following steps to complete the whole design. The main objectives of cross-sectional study include:

①To describe the distribution of health-related states and determinants in the population.

②To provide etiological clues and generate hypotheses for analytic studies.

③To establish some reference values to physiological or biochemical markers, or to conduct a screening for three levels of prevention.

④To evaluate effectiveness and efficiency of service for disease prevention and control.

3. 2. 3. 2　To Select the Study Population

According to the study objectives, the target population, which the final sampled population could represent and the survey conclusion could extrapolate, should be defined in a certain range of region, ethnicity or race. Subsequently, the composition unit of the target population should be classified and a sampling frame including some sampling units should be determined. The sampling unit often refers to an individual person, institution or entity. The target population provides the overall context and represents the collection of sampling units in which inferences and estimates are desired. Moreover, the selected populations for a cross-sectional study may have a higher prevalence of a disease, or higher probability of developing the disease.

3.2.3.3   To Select Survey Methods

As described above, survey methods should be selected with the aim of study as the reference. If the choice is a census, it is important to determine the scope of the census. If a sampling survey is adopted, the sampling method and implementation process must be determined. For a sample survey, the main goal is to obtain a representative sample from which one can infer the relevant data for the entire population. Also, human resources, organizational strength and budget should be involved in reaching a determinate certain survey.

3.2.3.4   To Select Variables or Factors

In cross-sectional studies, data on exposure (potential risk factors) and outcomes are collected simultaneously. The choice of exposure and outcome variables is based on the objectives of the study and on biological considerations. Generally, the considering factors include some contents about frequency index of disease, such as mortality, incidence, prevalence rate, disability, living quality, burden of disease, and etc. The data of demography, such as name, sex, nation, age, occupation, socio-economic status, degree of education, and address or telephone are also taken into consideration. The major contents include some correlated factors which devote to the disease in different degrees.

3.2.3.5   To Design Questionnaires

How the contents can be transformed into the information that we need? A questionnaire is generally designed to acquire information by a series of questions. There is no fixed format for questionnaires, and their contents should be chosen to make the instrument most applicable to the scientific objectives of the investigation, while also taking in account requirements for processing and analyzing the data. Questionnaires can include open and closed questions. Answers to an open question are not pre-specified and are provided in the subject's own words. Closed questions require the subject to choose from a list of options.

As the major tool of survey, the questionnaire wholly affects the validity and reliability of data. Good design of questionnaires requires skill. Questionnaires are useful for collecting information that may be difficult to obtain in any other way. Although designing a questionnaire seems simple, it is in fact rather difficult than we think. Whenever possible, use pretested questionnaires from the local or international organizations (such as the host MOH, WHO, DHS). Consequently, new questions can be developed with additional information. Pictures are useful for illustrating questions that are difficult to state in words or for illiterate data collectors. To develop complete questionnaires, the focus of group discussions can be used to develop the first draft.

Principles should be followed during questionnaire design:

①The survey should include relevant questions and exclude irrelevant items. Questionnaires should be short and concise. The required items should be considered as possible, and those non-correlated items should be excluded without hesitation.

②The questions should be expressed with common words to avoid misunderstanding and terminology should be neglected; particularly, the answer item should include all possible elements. Two short questions, each covering one point, are better than one long question which covers two points.

③Objective measures, especially for risk factors, are preferable, whenever possible. For example, we would ask "how many cigarettes do you smoke one day?" rather than "do you smoke cigarette?"

④The former questions would be easy to reply, those questions that need to comprehend should be arranged subsequently, and the susceptible questions are arranged lastly.

⑤Furthermore, a questionnaire is rarely finished one time, because usually it makes the questionnaire more applicable after several times of the pilot survey. Open questions are difficult to code. Therefore, some information-format code should be considered to make the inputting data more convenient.

Key steps for questionnaire design:

①Define indicators that meet the survey objectives, including the definition of cases and events.

②Identify the easiest method for assessing each indicator and develop questions which can produce the required information for each indicator. Decide whether to make the questions open-ended or closed-ended.

③Check each question against the survey objectives. Keep only those questions that provide the most essential information.

④Ensure each question is clear, simple, short, and easy to ask.

⑤Test new questions on dummy tables to confirm that they could assess the selected indicators.

⑥Translate the questionnaire into the local language and then translate it back to the original language to identify any mistakes.

⑦Ensure there is a logical flow of questions in each section. Begin with general questions and end with the more sensitive questions.

⑧Place instructions for the interviewers at the beginning of each section.

⑨Provide enough space between questions for recording responses.

⑩Pilot/try out the questionnaire and other survey instruments (e. g. , weighing scales, tape measures) in an area that is not to be surveyed. Check to ensure that no essential information has been left out and the interview is short (less than 20 minutes).

⑪Review the questionnaire and make final changes.

For example, one public health doctor designed a questionnaire to investigate the prevalence rate of diabetes in a certain population (Table 3.1).

Table 3.1   Example: Questionnaire for Diabetes Survey

Code: □-□□□

A   General Information

1. Name: first name _____ last name _____

2. Sex   ①male ②female   □

3. Birthday ____/____/_____ (mm/dd/yyyy)

4. Occupation ①worker ②farmer ③businessman ④staff ⑤unemployed ⑥else _____ □

5. Degree of Education

①illiteracy ②primary school ③middle school ④college and above   □

6. Did you get married?   ①yes ②no   □

7. How much did you spend on purchasing food per month (RMB)?   □

①<200   ②200~400   ③500~700   ④≥800

B   History of Disease

1. Did the doctor once tell you that you had got diabetes? ①yes   ②no   □

   If not, please jump to "C".

2. If yes, what time were you examined as a diabetes patient? ____/____/_____(mm/dd/yyyy)

3. And in what hospital did you receive the diagnosis?   □

①town hospital   ②county hospital   ③county hospital above

4. Did you take some drugs to control the level of blood sugar? ①yes   ②no   □

5. If yes, what the main kind of drug did you take? And how long?

①_____; _____ years   ②_____; _____ years

③_____; _____ years   ④_____; _____ years

C   Physical Examination

1. Height _____ cm   2. Weight _____ kg

3. Waist Circumference _____ cm   4. Hip Circumference _____ cm

5. Fast Glucose _____ mg/dl   6. Blood Pressure _____ / _____ mmHg (SBP/DBP)

Interview Date ____/____/_____ (mm/dd/yyyy)   **Signature** _____

In designing a questionnaire, sometimes extra items are added with a completely different wording of an existing question. These items called "sleepers" or "liar catchers" are supposed to provide with "internal validity" for some important questions. But if the responder realizes that he is being asked the same question twice he may elect to refuse to provide further answers.

3.2.3.6   To Collect Background Data

(1)Collection of the Background Data

The recent progress of the topic of the proceeding survey should be viewed broadly. Only according to the accomplished study, new ideas and reasonable considerations can be reached, which could show the survey feasibility. There are three ways to hold the background data. The first is to summarize self-experience, the second is to learn from other experts, and the third is to read literature about a similar topic.

(2)Measurement of Disease

The survey should make a generally accepted diagnostic criterion for the disease and the diagnostic technology should be simple, highly sensitive and easy to conduct. For some severe diseases and chronic uncured diseases, such as cancers and cirrhosis, the false positive rate should be lower, which is more important than higher sensitivity. This is different from clinical diagnosis.

(3)Measurement of Exposure

It is the main part for cross-sectional study to collect information on current and past levels of exposure. The exposure or the correlated factors should be defined distinctly, and the way to measure them should be described clearly. What time the exposure occurred, how long the exposure lasted and the different degree of exposure should be showed when we measure exposure information. As for smoking, the first question should be "have you smoked recently?". The definition of smoking is smoking for at least more than 6 months and smoking more than 20 cigarettes a week. The answer would be ①no, never, ②yes, ③ smoked formerly, and now have stopped smoking. The second question is "how many cigarettes do you smoke every day?", and the next question usually is "how old did you start smoking?" or "how many years have you smoked?", and sometimes, there is an additional question that is why you stop smoking.

(4)Means of Data Collecting or Variables Measurement

Means of variables measurement include face-to-face interview, mail interview, telephone interview, some special survey technology, etc. The means of examination measurement includes physical examination, experimental examination, etc.

(5)Request for Interviewers

The interviewers should be systematically trained and only those who have passed the strict training examination could conduct the interview. The interviewers should not induce the objects to respond so that less bias is produced.

3.2.3.7 Data Analysis

(1)The Description of Demographic Characteristics

A detailed description of the sample distribution according to gender, age, culture level, occupation, marital status, social and economic status, etc., provides an important picture of the study population and can be useful in comparison with other surveys.

(2)Reporting Disease Distribution Data

Data for the population can be grouped according to various personal characteristics such as gender, age, educational level, occupation, marital status, etc. Geographic characteristics may include distinctions between urban and rural, north and south, or according to administrative districts. Time characteristics may be presented according to the season, month or year.

(3)Associations Between Exposure and Diseases

In a cross-sectional study it is possible to calculate and report a prevalence ratio with its 95% confidence interval for associations between risk factors and diseases, and these estimates can be adjusted for the possible confounding effects of measures covariates.

3.2.4   Quality Control of Survey

The measures of quality control include:

①The sample selection should be randomized.

②A pilot survey should be carried out before the formal survey.

③The response rate should be higher than 80%—90%.

④The Interviewers should pass the uniform strict training.

⑤The methods of survey and examination should be standardized and stabilized.

⑥Repetition surveying or checking 5%—10% of the population.

⑦To crosscheck the correctness of data before and after inputting into the computer and arrange data orderly in order to make it reasonable to analyze.

⑧To control the bias.

Lastly, to report the main findings is the most important part of the study. The report should list the objectives, discuss what has been achieved and what has not and why. Reporting disadvantage in predictions will help those who are planning to do a similar survey avoid a similar mistake. Report the target number of subjects and the percentage response achieved. How this will affect the statistical power of the tests performed versus the power expected in the proposal. The last part of the report is the conclusions. What has been achieved? Are the results in line with the predictions? If not, clarify the reason why the difference occurs. Was any new hypothesis generated by the extra analysis performed? Is it necessary to perform another study to test these new hypotheses? In which way can these results be utilized by others?

3.3   Census and Sampling Survey

3.3.1   Census

It is called a census if researchers recruit and gather information from almost all members in a target population. A census is often considered as the best way to provide a comprehensive understanding of the health status in a population. However, it is not easy to count everyone, nor, does everyone want to be counted. Extraordinary efforts will be taken to get everyone surveyed.

3.3.3.1   Target of Census

A census is usually employed to describe the distribution of diseases in a population, or the health level of residents, or to establish some reference values to physiological or biochemical markers. For example, a census is regularly, nearly once per ten years, conducted to investigate the population composition of the whole country in China. Also, a census is used to conduct a screening for three levels of prevention of diseases, especially for early detection, early diagnosis and early treatment of patients, such as the married women who were examined by a Pap smear to test for cervical cancer as early as possible.

3.3.3.2 Principles of Census

①One primary aim of the census is to find all patients and treat them betimes.

②The prevalence rate of the disease should be high enough so that many of patients could be found.

③The diagnosis of the disease should be sensitive, specific, simple and convenient in the field.

④There should be enough manpower, fund, material, and equipment to detect patients and essential treatment should be considered.

3.3.3.3 Advantages of Census

①The census can provide an enormous resource bank of health information, which can exhibit a panorama of the health status and help find all the patients in a population and make it possible to treat them betimes.

②The epidemic character could be described roundly from the analysis of census data, and the inhabitants could acquire much more knowledge of disease prevention and control.

③The census can observe the relationships between multi-factors and a disease.

④There are less medical ethical problems in the census.

3.3.3.4 Disadvantages of Census

It is very expensive. The census is not befitting to those diseases with low prevalence rate and none availability of simple and convenient diagnosis technique in the field. It is not easy to control the quality because there are so many objects in the census. Inaccuracies may result if the personnel conducting the surveys are not properly trained.

3.3.2 Sampling Survey

3.3.2.1 Definition

The sampling survey is to select a specified number of persons from a finite population (sample, a subset of a population) to make inferences, on the basis of the sample data, about overall population quantities, such as the prevalence rate or other characteristics (Figure 3.3). Generally, a sampling survey is designed with the hope that it can be a representative of the entire population.

3.3.2.2 Basic Principle

In practice, a sample survey needs a representative sample for greater accuracy, and thus the sample should be randomly selected. Each individual unit (village, household or

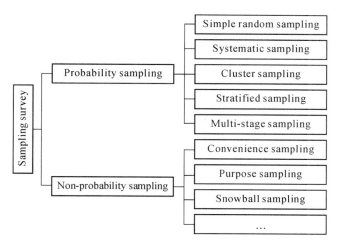

Figure 3. 3   Category of Sampling Survey

person) should have an equal chance of being included. And the sample size should be appropriately settled with precision (larger sample size, less measurement error) of the character of population inferred from a sample survey. For example, as an important supplement to the census, China sometimes conducts population sampling surveys in order to keep abreast of the latest population composition.

3.3.2.3   Method

Sampling is defined as the selection of a specified number of persons in a population for study with the hope that they are *representative*, i. e. , the characteristics of the sampled population (study population) are similar to the population from which it is drawn (reference population). Sampling can be divided into probability sampling and non-probability sampling (Figure 3. 3, detailed information about non-probability sampling can be referred to other epidemiology textbooks).

In probability sampling, every person in the target population has the same known (and non-zero) chance of being included in the survey. It allows investigators to form conclusions about a reference population based on information collected only from a subset of the population. Probability sampling, therefore, enables the collection of reliable information at a minimal cost. Results from these surveys can also be compared with results of similar surveys performed in another time, place or population.

The followings are probability sampling methods:

(1)Simple Random Sampling (SRS)

Firstly, the sampling unit (person, household, village, community, etc.) from which the sample is to be drawn is listed, which is often called a sample frame. Then the required number of units are randomly selected from the sampling frame by drawing lots or using random numbers (either a table of random numbers from textbooks or the module of random numbers of computer software, e. g. , Microsoft Excel or R).

This method is more likely to produce a representative sample, but it can be expensive and difficult to make a sampling frame where a population is scattered. Moreover, it is also quite laborious to accomplish a sampling survey with SRS, as the sample units may be too scattered.

(2)Systematic Sampling

It begins by randomly selecting the starting unit, in order to fulfil statistical requirements in systematic selection. The next sampling units are systematically selected by adding a certain number "n" (e. g. , 10, 20, 50 depending on the sample size relative to the total population) to the starting unit.

A systematic sample can be drawn without an initial listing (e. g. , choose from a line of people, the registry number of outpatients' clinic, or according to the time patients enter a clinic).

(3)Cluster Sampling

Cluster sampling begins with a list of clusters, and clusters can be communities or administrative subdivisions (e. g. , sublocation, village, zone, plot, class, school, etc.). For the first stage, a certain number of clusters are randomly selected, based on the cumulative frequency distribution of a population. For the second stage, a specific number of sub-units are randomly selected within each selected cluster. Comparatively speaking, cluster sampling is much easier to implement than SRS. But in order to ensure the data precision, more clusters and smaller sample size per each cluster are needed.

(4)Stratified Sampling

First, populations are stratified into several strata by the character of areas, ages, genders, etc. Then the subjects are selected using a random sampling method in each stratum.

(5)Multi-Stage Sampling

The multi-stage sampling is composed of several levels of random sampling (one for each stage). A multi-stage sampling is often employed in a large-scale investigation (e. g. , a nationwide study) which is not convenient for direct selecting study subjects. For example, sampling from a population of pupils is shown in Figure 3. 4.

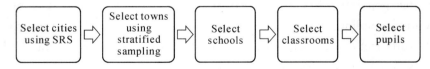

Figure 3. 4　Example of Multi-Stage Sampling

3.3.2.4　Sample Size Estimation

In general, the larger the sample, the more reliable the estimated parameters of the entire population will be. Therefore, the size of a selected sample should be large enough to give reliable estimates. But too large sample size would waste limited resources. Two parameters should be considered when estimating the sample sizes: the precision and prevalence. If the precision is high, permitted measurement error should be small, and thus a larger sample size is needed. If the prevalence of disease is low, a larger sample size is needed.

The following formulas can be used for calculating the minimum sample sizes for SRS. Formula(3. 1) for numerical data:

$$N = \left(\frac{Z_{1-\alpha/2} S}{d} \right)^2 \qquad (3.1)$$

N—size of the sample; Z—level of statistical certainty chosen, or confidence interval: $Z_{1-0.05/2} = 1.96$, $Z_{1-0.10/2} = 1.68$; S—the evaluated value of σ; d—tolerance/allowable deviation (the difference between the sample mean and total mean), half of the confidence interval.

Note: Confidence interval is the range of values obtained from the sample survey between which we are 95% confident that the true value in the overall population lies.

Formula(3. 2) for categorical data (estimating sample size for simple random or systematic sampling):

$$N = \left(\frac{Z_{1-\alpha/2}^2 PQ}{d^2} \right) \qquad (3.2)$$

N—size of the sample; Z—level of statistical certainty chosen, or confidence interval, $Z_{1-0.05/2} = 1.96$, $Z_{1-0.10/2} = 1.68$; d—degree of accuracy desired = half of the confidence interval; P—estimated level/prevalence/coverage rate being investigated; $Q = 1 - P$

How to estimate the sample size of cluster sampling? The exact size of the clusters is often unknown at the time of sampling-need weighted analysis. In practice, calculating sample size requires considering the balance between precision and cost, and individuals within a cluster tend to be more alike than those in different clusters resulting in larger standard errors for estimates. Loss of precision must be anticipated at the design stage by increasing the sample size. Thus, one may approximately double the sample size in order to maintain the same degree of precision as SRS, because this type of sampling has some degree of selection bias. Also, sample size tables in standard statistics textbooks can be used to determine the actual sample size needed.

3. 3. 2. 5 Advantage and Disadvantage

The sampling survey can save manpower, material resources and time, and the accuracy is great. But the design, implement and data analysis of sampling survey are complex, and thus it isn't suitable for the data with a great variation or the disease with low prevalence rate. Differences between census and sampling survey are listed in Table 3. 2.

Table 3. 2   Differences Between Census and Sampling Survey

Item	Census	Sampling Survey
Participant	Whole target population	Sample
Strength	No sampling error	The workload is small; More detailed and complete information can be obtained; Because the scope of the investigation is small, it can save time, manpower and material resources.
Weakness	Heavy workload; greater consumption of manpower, material and financial resources; difficult to obtain detailed health information; not suitable for investigating diseases with low prevalence	Unavoidable sampling error; more complex design; not applicable to diseases with low prevalence and excessive variability

3. 4   Case Report and Case Survey

Case reports are detailed descriptions of a few patients or clinical cases (frequently, just one sick person) with an unusual disease or complication, uncommon combinations of diseases, an unusual or misleading semiology, cause, or outcome (maybe a surprising recovery). They often are preliminary observations that are later refuted. They cannot estimate disease frequency or risk (e. g. , for lack of a valid denominator). Alternatives are available for completing the clinical picture. Many problems worthy of investigation in medicine are first identified by observations at the bedside. Indeed, case reports may thoughtfully integrate clinical, anatomopathological, genetic, pathophysiological, occupational, or biochemical information and reasoning; they may thus build a sound mechanistic or pragmatic hypothesis and set the foundation for (micro)biological studies and for larger clinical and epidemiological studies. They may also raise a thoughtful suspicion of a new adverse drug event and are an important means of surveillance for rare clinical events.

In 1962, some articles were published to report cases of Congenital Disorders (e. g. , both thumbs underdeveloped and considerable deformity of both forearms; both legs twisted and shortened). These pieces of literature discovered one common phenomenon that nearly all mothers had a history of taking thalidomide during pregnancy and thus revealed the possible relationship between thalidomide and congenital disorders.

The case series is a collection of subjects (usually patients) with common characteristics used to describe some clinical, pathophysiological, or operational aspects of a disease, treatment, exposure, or diagnostic procedure. Some are similar to the larger case reports and share their virtues. The number of subjects does not attenuate the limitations of the design. A case series does not include a comparison group and is often based on prevalent cases and a convenience sample.

3.5   Ecological Study

3.5.1   Definition

The ecological study is an investigation of the distribution of health and its determinants between groups of individuals.

Different from a cross-sectional study, the unit of analysis in an ecological study is a population. Ecological studies explore the correlation between disease rates or ratios in different population groups and estimate average exposures in groups (locations or time periods) rather than individuals. For example, they may correlate death rates across cities or towns with estimates of exposure, such as factory emissions in a given geographic area, proximity to waste sites, or air or water pollution levels (e. g. , $PM_{2.5}$ and PM_{10}). The geographical information system (GIS) is a useful tool that improves the ability of ecological studies to determine a link between health data and environmental exposure.

Often the information about disease and exposure is abstracted from published statistics, or directly obtained from routine work of a government department (e. g. , Center for Disease Control and Prevention or environmental protection departments) and therefore does not require expensive or time-consuming data collection. The populations compared may be defined in various ways, e. g. , by locations (countries or cities) or time periods.

3.5.2   Category

3.5.2.1   Ecological Comparison Study

Disease rates (Y) and exposures (X) are measured in each of a series of populations and their relationship is examined. Whether eating spicy food is good for health has always been an interesting topic. Now we design an ecological study to discuss this topic. We collect pepper sales information from the commercial supervisory authority in each city and disease incidence data from the health bureau, and then divide cities into three groups, according to the pepper consumption (risk factor, X), and then compare the diseases incidence, morbidity and mortality of disease (such as gastric ulcer morbidity, all-cause mortality). Now, let's change to a simpler and more intuitive description, such as making a scatter plot of pepper sales and disease A incidence in each city. If the graph is similar to Figure 3.5, the incidence of disease A is high in cities with larger sales of pepper, but low in cities with smaller sales of pepper, then we can make a conclusion that pepper may be positively related to the incidence of disease A. These investigations and analyses can help us to deepen our understanding on this topic.

3.5.2.2   Ecological Time Trends Study

The ecological time-trend study investigates the temporal relationship between the fluc-

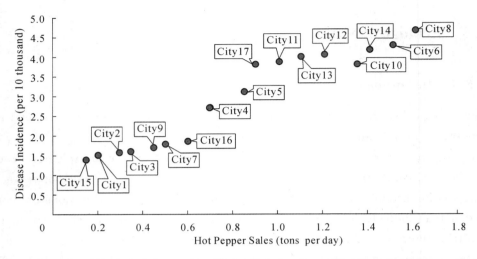

Figure 3.5   Example of Ecological Comparison Study (Relationship of Hot Pepper and Disease Incidence)
  Note: All data in the figure was simulated.

tuations of average exposure level (or intervention implemented) and frequency changes of disease in a population. Many diseases show remarkable differences in incidence over time (e. g. , air pollution and diseases incidence). For example, one research collected registry data from a hospital and concurrent air pollution monitoring data from the air pollution monitoring station in a city. Data analysis revealed that the number of outpatients with respiratory diseases increased by 0. 26% among children with an increase of $10\mu g/m^3$ in contemporaneous daily $PM_{2.5}$ concentration.

Rates of acute infection can vary appreciably over a few days, but epidemics of chronic disorders such as lung cancer and coronary heart disease evolve over decades. If the trend of disease incidence correlates with the changes in a community's environment or life style (e. g. , reduction of smoking or alcohol abuse rate, promotion of smartphones and gradual improvement of hygienic conditions), then the trends may provide important clues to etiology. Recent statistics revealed a continuous drop in cancer death rate and incidence rate in the US. Suppose that we draw a scatter plot with annual cancer incidence rate and annual smoking rate and find a concurrent decline tendency of these two rates (or we examined this with a regression model and found a positive association between annual smoking rate and cancer incidence rate), we may hypothesize that smoking cessation policy may serve as a possible cause of the decline in cancer incidence. We can also analyze the relationship of pepper and disease A with a design of ecological time-trend study. We can also collect annual pepper sales and disease incidence just in one city, and then draw two lines (Figure 3. 6) of pepper sales and disease A incidence. As time goes by, the dietary structure of citizen has changed tremendously and the sales of chili peppers have kept increasing year by year. Meanwhile, the incidence of disease A has also increased gradually. We can also make an etiologic hypothesis that chili peppers may be related to disease A.

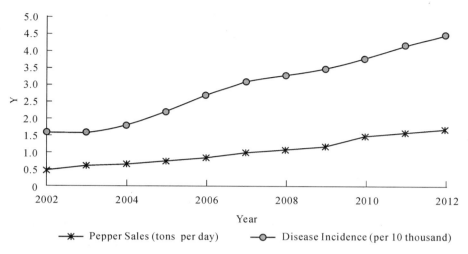

Figure 3.6   Example of Ecological Time-Trend Study (Relationship of Pepper Sales and Disease Incidence)
Note: All data in the figure was simulated.

3.5.2.3   Mixed Study

In fact, comparison study and trends study are often combined to investigate the relationship between exposure and disease. Mixed study may be conducted to investigate the fluctuations of chronic noncommunicable diseases (e. g. , diabetes mellitus, hypertension, cancer) of residents in different cities over several decades, which will provide more useful information of the relationship of chronic diseases and lifestyle (e. g. , smoking, Excessive drinking, internet addiction) or environment factors (e. g. , air or water pollution, climate change).

3.5.3   Applications

①To offer clues for the cause of a disease.

②To provide affirmation or negate substantial evidence for the causal hypothesis which has been generated.

③To help evaluate the effect of interventional or field trials.

④To explore the effect of exposure without much fluctuations or not easy to detect individually on the disease.

⑤To apply for disease surveillance.

Many useful observations have emerged from geographical analyses. One typical application is to look for geographical correlations between disease incidence or mortality and the prevalence of risk factors. However, attention is needed in the interpretation of ecological studies. Bias may occur if ascertainment of disease or exposure, or both, differs from one place to another. Like geographical studies, an analysis of secular trends may be biased by differences in the ascertainment of disease. As health services have been improved, diagnostic criteria and techniques have changed. Furthermore, whereas in geographical studies the differences are accessible to current inquiry, validating secular changes is more difficult as it depends on observations made and often scantily recorded many years ago. Nevertheless, the reality-if not the true size-of secular trends can often be established with reasonable certainty.

3.5.4　Strengths and Weaknesses

3.5.4.1　Strengths

①It is quick, inexpensive (often based on routine work or published data), and does not require manpower and time-consuming data collection.

②Provide clues to help formulate a hypothesis for a disease with unknown etiology.

③Exposure and disease are measured and compared at the area or time periods level, not individuals, especially applicable to evaluating the effectiveness of interventions implemented at the group level, and to exploring the correlation between disease and exposure of individuals with small variations within the population.

④A simple correlation coefficient is used to measure the association.

3.5.4.2　Weaknesses

①It could not provide accurate information about the relationship between risk factors and diseases in individuals. The ecological fallacy should not be ignored when the real individual exposure is not equal to the average population level, or the exposed population does not correspond to the patient population.

②The second weakness is its inability to control for confounding factors.

③Similar to other descriptive studies, the ecological study cannot confirm the causal inference between exposure and disease, because whether exposure occurred before the disease cannot be ascertained.

(Wang Ziyun, Shen Chong, Zhao Jinshun)

Exercise

Chapter 4　Cohort Study

The objective of a cohort study is to measure and usually to compare the incidence of disease in one or more cohorts. This chapter is organized as follows: firstly, an introduction of cohort studies including main conceptual features and historical development of cohort studies is given; secondly, the key concerns of cohort studies including the selection of the studied population and the important question of how to determine the exposure and measure the exposure events, and basic concepts regarding data analysis in cohort studies are described; lastly, the specific types of bias in the framework of a cohort study, the ethical issues, advantages and disadvantages regarding cohort studies will be discussed.

4.1　Introduction

4.1.1　Definition of a Cohort Study

The word "cohort" came from Latin "cohors". A cohort was originally defined as one of the ten divisions of a legion in the Roman army consisting of 300 to 600 men. The most common application of cohort today is to describe a demographic group of people, especially those having common characteristics. For example, a birth cohort is defined as the component of the population born during the same period of time, thus, sharing a common life event. In this case, its characteristics (e. g. , causes of death and those still living) can be ascertained as it enters successive time and age periods. Currently, the meaning of "cohort" has been broadened to designate a group of people who share a common experience or condition. In the cohort study of epidemiology, a cohort is used to describe a designated group of persons who are followed or traced over a period of time. The cohort study (also named as concurrent study, follow-up study, incidence study, longitudinal study, panel study, or prospective study), is an analytic epidemiological study in which subsets of a defined population can be identified who are, have been, or in the future may be exposed or not exposed, or exposed in different degrees, to a factor or factors hypothesized to influence the occurrence of a given disease or other health-related events (outcomes). The main feature of a cohort study is to observe a large number of subjects over a long period, by comparing with incidence rates in groups with different exposure levels. As the alternative terms of a cohort study (e. g. , follow-up study, longitudinal study, or prospective study) suggested, the essential feature of the method is to observe the population for a sufficient time to generate reliable incidence or mortality rates.

The design of a cohort study is illustrated in Figure 4.1. In brief, both a group of individuals exposed to a putative risk factor (exposed group) and a group of individuals who are unexposed to this risk factor (control group) are followed over time (e. g. , months, years) to compare the incidence of the disease. Although only two groups are illustrated in Figure 4.1, the design may include more than two groups. The relative risk is usually used to assess whether exposure and disease are causally linked.

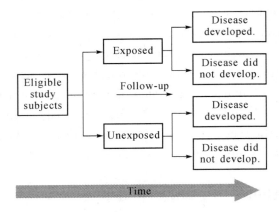

Figure 4. 1   Design of a Cohort Study

4. 1. 2   A Brief History of Cohort Studies

Cohort studies have been used for over a century to investigate the causes of diseases and to establish links between risk factors and health outcomes. During the early days of epidemiology, it has been used as a powerful tool to study a variety of exposures, including microbial infections, nutritional factors, occupational exposures, and lifestyle factors.

4. 1. 2. 1   Cohort Studies of Infectious Diseases

The London cholera epidemic study conducted by John Snow is a very classical example of a cohort study of infectious diseases. In the mid-19th century, due to the large influx of people and a lack of proper sanitary services, the Soho district of London faced a problem with filth. There were many cesspools with night soil located in the cellars which were all dumped into the River Thames, thus increasing the filthy streams which flowed through southern England. This action contaminated the water supply, leading to the risk of cholera outbreak; but it was not recognized during that time. Eventually, a major outbreak of cholera struck the Soho district on 31st August 1854, and over the next three days, 127 people on or nearby the Broad Street died. Over the following week, three-quarter of the residents had left the area. By 10th September, cholera took 500 people's lives and thereby drawn the attention of the Registrar General as they reported the possibility that differences in the water supply were associated with the mortality of cholera across sections of London. The two different water companies (the Lambeth and the Southwark & Vauxhall) were responsible for the households' water supplying within various regions of London. One important different feature was that the two companies differed in the location of the water intake. The Lambeth company had moved water intake upstream from the sewage discharge point in 1849, while the Southwark & Vauxhall still obtained water downstream of the sewage discharge point. Dr. Snow started the investigation and classified households according to their exposure to the two different water sources and found out a substantial difference in cholera mortality, which was 315 cholera deaths per 10,000 households served by the Southwark & Vauxhall versus 37 cholera deaths per 10,000 households served by Lambeth companies. Cohort studies have been a useful tool in the investigation of various infectious diseases. For instance, McCray (1986) used a cohort design to quantitate prospectively the risk to health care workers, who were exposed to blood and body fluids of patients with acquired immunodeficiency syndrom (AIDS).

4.1.2.2   Cohort Studies of Nutritional Factors

Pellagra is a type of vitamin deficiency disease, most frequently caused by a chronic lack of intake of niacin (vitamin B3) in the diet. Its dermatological effects were firstly described by Gaspar Casal in Spain in 1735. Pellagra was endemic in the southeast of the US in the late 19th and early 20th century. Dr. Joseph Goldberger employed a variety of epidemiological approaches, including cohort study methods, to study Pellagra. He investigated the dietary exposures of households related to the occurrence of pellagra and finally indicated that a cornmeal subsistence diet was associated with the increased risk of pellagra. Subsequent trials further showed that pellagra did not transmit from person to person like most infectious diseases, and could be actually prevented by the "pellagra-preventive factor" which was later determined to be niacin.

4.1.2.3   Cohort Studies of Occupational Exposures

Occupational epidemiology is another classical field with many applications of cohort studies. Application of the cohort studies has been a powerful tool in the identification of many occupational hazards and quantification of associated risks. For example, occupational cohorts worked as a tool to study the association between exposure to dyes and urinary bladder cancer, the association between the exposure to mustard gas and respiratory cancer, and exposure to benzene and leukemia. Ulvestad and colleagues implemented a cohort study on members of the Norwegian Trade Union of insulation workers who were hired between 1930 and 1975, demonstrating relative increases in the risk of mesothelioma and lung cancer when compared with the general population.

4.1.2.4   Cohort Studies of Lifestyle Factors

Lifestyle exposures, including physical activity, tobacco smoking, and alcohol consumption, have attracted the attention of epidemiologists. Morris et al. (1953) demonstrated that British bus drivers had about double risks of heart disease in comparison to the conductors who were more active and went up and down the stairs to collect tickets. Around 1950, results of several case-control studies had been published demonstrating an association between lung cancer and cigarette smoking, including those from Doll and Hill (1950). However, at that time, some argued that smoking might be a factor in the development of a disease. Thus, one of the landmark studies was the cohort study that Doll and Hill initiated in 1951 by collecting data on tobacco use via a questionnaire among British physicians. Through the cohort study, they demonstrated a 10-fold increased risk of lung cancer death in smokers compared to non-smokers (Doll and Peto, 1976).

4. 1. 2. 5   Cohort Studies of Non-communicable Diseases

Cardiovascular disease (CVD) is a leading cause of death and serious illness in the United States. During the middle of the 20th century, little was known about the causes of heart disease and stroke, but the death rates for CVD had been steadily increasing since the beginning of the century. In 1948, the Framingham Heart Study (FHS) initiated a novel project to identify the common factors or characteristics that contributed to CVD. The study followed a large group of participants who had not yet developed overt symptoms of CVD or suffered a heart attack or stroke for a long period of time. In 1948, the researchers recruited 5,209 men and women between the ages of 30 and 62 from the town of Framingham, Massachusetts, US, and began the first round of extensive physical examinations and lifestyle interviews that they would later analyze for common patterns related to CVD development. Since 1948, the participants came back after two years for an examination consisting of a detailed medical history, physical examination, and laboratory tests. In 1971, the study enrolled a second-generation cohort, 5,124 of the original participants' adult children and their spouses, to participate in similar examinations. The second examination of the offspring cohort occurred eight years after the first examination, and subsequent examinations have been performed approximately every four years. On April 2002, the study entered a new phase: the enrollment of the third generation of participants, the grandchildren of the original cohort. The first examination of the third-generation study was completed in July 2005 and involved 4,095 participants. Thus, the FHS has evolved into a prospective, community-based, three generation family study. The FHS cohort study identified major CVD risk factors, including high blood pressure, high blood cholesterol, smoking, obesity, diabetes, and physical inactivity, as well as a great deal of valuable information on the effects of related factors, for instance, blood triglyceride and HDL cholesterol levels, ages, genders, and psychosocial issues. In the past 50 years, the study has published approximately 1,200 articles in leading medical journals. The landmark CVD risk factor studies have become an integral part of the modern medical curriculum and have led to the development of effective treatment and preventive strategies in clinical practice.

4. 1. 3   Prospective Versus Retrospective Cohort Studies

Cohort studies may be classified as either prospective or retrospective (Figure 4. 2).

4. 1. 3. 1   Prospective Cohort Study

A prospective cohort study is also called a concurrent cohort study, where the subjects have been followed up over time and the outcomes of interest are recorded. It is carried out from the present to the future and can be tailored to collect specific exposures; but there may be a long wait for events to occur, particularly when the outcome of certain interest is associated with old age. Prospective cohort studies thus can be expensive to carry out and are prone to high rates of loss to follow up, although these can be overcome by incorporating a dynamic study design. The prospective study is especially important for research on the etiology of diseases and disorders.

4. 1. 3. 2   Retrospective Cohort Study

A retrospective cohort study is also called a historical cohort study. One main feature is that in retrospective cohort studies, both the exposure and outcome have already occurred at the outset of the study. The investigators must reconstruct the historical experience of the participants from available records or from interviews and questionnaires. One advantage of retrospective cohort studies is that the information is available immediately, and moreover, this type of study is less time-consuming and less costly than a prospective cohort study. However, it is more susceptible to the effects of bias. For example, the exposure may have occurred some years ago, and information on exposure and confounding variables may be unavailable, inadequate or difficult to collect.

4. 1. 3. 3   Ambidirectional Cohort Study

A cohort study may also be ambidirectional, meaning that there is a coexistence of retrospective and prospective phases in the study. Ambidirectional studies are less common than pure prospective or retrospective studies, but they are conceptually consistent with and share elements of the advantages and disadvantages of both types of studies.

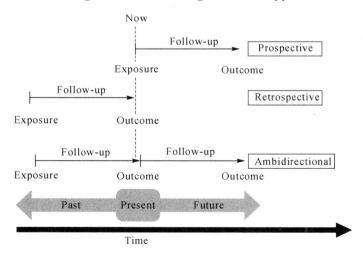

Figure 4. 2   Schematic Diagram of Prospective, Retrospective, and Ambidirectional Cohort Study

4. 1. 4   Nested Case-Control Study

A nested case-control study is a specific type of cohort study. The study design is often used in case the exposure of interest is difficult or expensive to obtain and when the outcome is rare. Utilizing data previously collected from a large cohort study can avoid the time and cost of initializing a new case-control study. In this case, if the measurement is only needed for the covariate in as many participants as necessary, the cost and effort of exposure assessment then are reduced. This benefit is obvious when the covariate of interest is biological, as assessments of gene expression profiling are expensive and the quantity of blood samples for such analysis is often with limited availability, thus making it a valuable resource.

For example, 91,523 women in the Nurses' Health Study who did not have cancer were enrolled and followed up for 14 years, and of which 2,341 had developed breast cancer by 1993. Several researchers have used standard cohort analyses to explore the precursors to breast cancer, e. g. , utilizing the hormonal contraceptives, which is a covariate easily measured among all of the participants in the cohort. If the research question is now to explore the association between gene expression and breast cancer incidence, it would be expensive and even uneconomical to assay all blood specimen of 89,000 women without breast cancer. In this case, one may consider to assay all of the cases, and at the same time, for selecting a certain number of women from the risk set of participants who have not yet developed breast cancer. The risk set is often restricted to those participants who are matched to the case on variables such as age, which reduces the variability of effect estimates. The number of controls depends on the rarity of the cases and the complexity of the measures of exposure, and frequently for each case 1—4 controls are selected.

4. 2   Design

4. 2. 1   Selection of Cohort Population

Regarding the selection of the study population, the cohort study aims to select participants who are identical with the exception of their exposure status. Ideally, all study participants in a cohort study, including exposed and unexposed, must be free of the outcome at the baseline and have the potential to develop the outcome in the future.

Both scientific and feasible considerations need to be given when the researchers are in the phase to select participants to form the study population in a cohort study. For common exposures, a general population cohort is feasible since it enables internal comparisons of exposure status and the population can be motivated and easy to follow up. For rare exposures, the cohort may be defined by geography or environmental exposure, or the cohort could be defined by specific occupation, e. g. , asbestos workers.

4. 2. 1. 1   Select the Exposure Group

(1) General Population

For common exposures, like tobacco smoking and alcohol drinking, a sufficiently large number of exposed individuals can often be identified by sampling from the general population. For example, gestational diabetes or hypertension during pregnancy are common exposures. A general population of pregnant women could be used to construct the cohort.

(2) Population with Specific Exposures

For rare exposures, like those related to specific occupations or environmental factors, it is more efficient to select subjects from a group of the specific population. For example, in a cohort study aiming to evaluate whether *in vitro* fertilization is a risk factor for the developmental disability in the offspring, sampling exposed subjects from an infertility clinic would be more reasonable rather than sampling from the general population. The benefit of selecting a population with special exposure is that it makes it possible to recruit sufficient numbers of exposed individuals in a reasonable time period. Also, subjects with specific exposures are more likely to clearly report the exposure than the general population. For example, conducting a cohort study among a group of blue-collar workers to evaluate the relationship between physical activity and the risk of coronary heart disease has clear advantages in terms of reduced sample size, accurate ascertainment of exposure, high levels of exposure, and ease of following to determine outcomes of interest. Moreover, utilizing a specific exposure cohort may permit evaluation of a rare outcome that would otherwise require an excessively large number of individuals.

4. 2. 1. 2   Select Control Group

Feasibility considerations for the unexposed group are similar to those for the exposed group. The unexposed group must be accessible for enrolment into the study and for follow-up. Controls should be selected from the source population where the cases come from. One important principle of selecting controls is that controls should be similar to the exposed group in important aspects, except without the exposure. The unexposed group can come from either internal or external sources.

(1) Internal Comparisons

Internal comparisons are most desirable. In a particular population, individuals were segregated by themselves (or through interventions) into different exposure status. For example, in a cohort study, 138 patients with HIV-associated Kaposi's sarcoma were divided into two groups: those with oral lesions and those with cutaneous lesions. The study revealed that the presence of oral lesions (the exposure) had a poorer prognosis.

(2) External Comparison Group

If internal controls are not available, researchers need to identify a comparison group somewhere else. For cohort studies using a specific exposure group, it is usually difficult to identify a portion of the cohort for comparison that can safely be assumed to be unexposed.

The principal is that the external comparison group should have similar characteristics with the exposed group in factors that may be related to the disease such as gender, geography, ethnic/racial composition, or other factors. It is important to guarantee that information obtained from the external comparison group is comparable with the exposed population.

(3) General Population

Occasionally, the occurrence of outcome in the exposed population is compared with the occurrence in the general population. This is particularly practical when members of the general population are unlikely to be exposed to the study factor, for example, occupational exposures. The advantage of using a selected comparison group is that it will probably be similar to the exposed cohort with regard to potential confounding factors. Moreover, potential confounders can be obtained and controlled in the analysis. However, the general population may not be comparable with those in the exposed group. For example, follow-up for the occurrence of disease may be more (or less) complete than for the exposed study group, which may lead to biased conclusions. Furthermore, if the exposed and unexposed groups are chosen from different time periods, medical care or other factors may differ between the groups in a way. A particular consideration pertains to occupational cohorts because people who are employed tend to be healthier than those who are not, and the general population includes people who are unable to work due to illness and disability. Accordingly, rates of disease and death measured among the general population are almost always higher than those of a population of factory workers. This phenomenon, termed the "healthy worker effect", may lead to the underestimated excess risk associated with a particular occupation in comparison with the general population.

(4) Multiple Comparison Groups

Sometimes it may be useful to have multiple comparison groups, especially when no single group appears sufficiently similar to the exposed cohort to ensure the validity of the comparison. In such circumstances, study results will be more convincing if different comparison groups are used and a similar association is observed.

(5) Other Issues

Cohort studies are often conducted among groups specifically chosen for their ability to facilitate the collection of relevant information, e. g. , members of medical professions, military veterans, students or alumni of particular universities, or residents of well-defined communities. These groups offer logistic advantages to the investigator, including the availability of regularly updated addresses, a mechanism for periodic follow-up, and the provision of complete medical and employment records.

4. 2. 2 Measure Exposures

4. 2. 2. 1 Definition of Exposure

Exposure is the variable whose causal effect is to be estimated. Common examples of exposures assessed by epidemiological studies include environmental factors, lifestyle factors, socioeconomic status, working conditions, medical treatments, or genetic traits. Exposures may be either harmful or beneficial, or even both (e. g. , if an immunizable disease is circulating, exposure to immunizing agents helps most recipients but may harm those with adverse reactions to the vaccine).

Cohort studies need a very clear definition of exposure at the beginning. This definition sometimes involves quantifying the exposure by degree, rather than just yes or no. For example, the minimum exposure to tobacco smoking might be defined as 14 cigarettes per day. Definition of exposure levels in this way can result in three groups—e. g. , nonsmokers, light smokers, and heavy smokers. Levels of exposure are measured for each individual at baseline of the study and then assessed during the period of follow-up.

A particular issue needed to be carefully concerned in cohort studies is whether participants in the control group are truly unexposed. For example, participants in the control group may start smoking during the follow-up period, or they may fail to report exposure status correctly. Similarly, those in the exposed group may change their behaviors in relation to exposure during the follow-up period.

4. 2. 2. 2   Methods to Obtain Exposure Information

In cohort studies, methods used to ascertain exposure vary from one study to another. Information on exposure status may be obtained from medical records, questionnaires, interviews, environment surveillance, or physical examination. Sometimes, in order to obtain adequate information on exposure, different sources of data may be used in combination in one cohort study.

(1) History Records

Using existing records has several advantages. First, information available for a high proportion of the study subjects is relatively inexpensive to obtain. In addition, since the data were recorded prior to the occurrence of the outcomes, the exposure information is unlikely to be biased by the outcomes.

(2) Interviews

Exposures in existing records may be insufficient to address specific research questions and lack information on potential confounders. Thus, interviews and questionnaires completed by study subjects or by proxy respondents, are often used to collect information on exposure and potential confounding factors. Quality of the interview data depends on the participants' ability to report details of the information. The stigma associated with certain exposures, such as alcohol or drug use, may have an influence on the response willingness of study subjects. It is therefore especially important to ensure that information is obtained in a comparable and unbiased manner for all participants.

(3) Physical Examination

A medical history may not always provide adequate information for some exposures or characteristics of interest, such as blood pressure or serum cholesterol levels. In this case, physical examination and/or laboratory test may be necessary. A series of biomarkers can be used to estimate exposure levels.

(4) Environment Monitoring

In case of investigation of certain occupational and environmental exposures, adequate information cannot be obtained from the sources mentioned above. In this case, the measurement of the air or water in a particular location can provide exposure data. The direct measurement may be possible for the evaluation of present or future exposures, but it may be problematic in situations where the exposure of interest has already occurred before the initiation of the study.

4.2.2.3　Issues Need to Be Considered

In many cohort studies, a single classification of exposure is made for each individual at the time when they enter into the study. However, exposure levels can change during the long-term follow-up period. For example, individuals may cease smoking, change jobs, or alter their dietary habits. Similarly, new equipment or working procedures being introduced to the workplace may increase or reduce the level of exposure of all workers in a single plant or an entire industry. Changes that diminish or increase exposure will tend to result in an underestimated or overestimated association between exposure and disease. Therefore, many cohort studies are designed to allow for periodic re-examination or repeated investigation of the members to acquire new information. During the analyses, the total length of exposure, changes in exposure status, and the reasons for these changes can be taken into account.

4.2.3　Follow Up

In any cohort study, no matter retrospective or prospective, ascertainment of outcome data involves tracing or following study participants from the time of exposure to the future to determine whether participants develop the health outcomes. Failure to obtain or collecting such information on a greater proportion of individuals in either the exposed or unexposed group is a major potential source of bias. A great deal of cost and time is required to ensure follow-up of cohort members and to update measures of exposures and confounders, in addition to monitoring participants' health outcomes. The failure to collect outcome data for cohort members will affect the validity of study results.

Cohort studies are usually conducted over a long period of time; thus, they are prone to follow-up bias. The follow-up process of the study, therefore, requires careful planning and implementation. It may be necessary to follow up at regular intervals or investigate only at the end of the study. Therefore, an agreement needs to be reached on how often follow-up should be taken. If the disease of interest has a long latent period, a long follow-up period will be needed. Researchers also need to consider that subjects may move away, die, or be lost to follow up in other ways. Therefore, a strategy for tracing subjects should be carefully planned. The required length of follow-up, or the interval that elapses between the definition of exposure status and ascertainment of the outcome, depends on the length of the latency period for the outcomes of interest. Outcomes such as acute infections have a latency period of just days to weeks between exposure and diagnosis, while congenital malformations and spontaneous abortions may require a few months to a year of observation. In contrast, chronic diseases like cancer and coronary heart diseases have very long latent periods and thus require decades to follow-up.

The loss to follow-up is problematic in most cohort studies and often leads to bias. Dropouts are not random events. If the likelihood of dropping out is related to the exposure or outcome, then the results can be biased, with the association between exposure and outcome being either over-estimated or under-estimated. For example, if people are suffering side effects from a particular drug during the follow-up period, they may drop out. In this case, the drug may look better than it actually is. To control the follow-up bias, it is better to select a stable population, motivate them to participate, and contact and trace them regularly. The analysis of data must include a comparison of risk factors between individuals who remain in the study and those who have dropped out. If the loss to follow-up is not considered, the reliability of study conclusions may be questioned.

4.2.4   Measure Disease Outcomes

Outcomes must be defined in advance and should be clear, specific and measurable. The outcome can be measured with records, interviews or examinations. One important principle is that the method used to ascertain outcomes must be identical for both exposed and control groups.

The sources of outcome data for a cohort study depend on the available resources and particular diseases of interest. The approach used to obtain outcome information may range from routine surveillance and death certificates to periodic questionnaires and health examinations for study participants of the cohort. The adequacy of death certificates for determining the cause-specific mortality depends on the particular disease under investigation and the setting in which death occurred. There is a potential bias in collecting or interpreting data from death records, especially when the records are vague and incomplete, or when the abstractor is also aware of a participant's exposure status. Therefore, investigators often look for additional confirmatory information from autopsies, physician or hospital records. For nonfatal endpoints, outcome data can be obtained from physicians' records, hospital discharge logs, population-based disease registries, or health insurance records. Investigators can also obtain data directly from the participants. The adequacy of self-reported diagnoses depends on the particular disease of interest. To reduce the potential bias due to the individual awareness of the hypothesis under investigation, information from hospital records or pathology reports are often accessed to confirm the information reported on questionnaires.

4.2.5   Estimate Disease Risk Associated with Exposure

The basic data analysis of a cohort study involves the calculation of incidence rates of a specified outcome among the cohort under investigation. These rates can be compared for those exposed and unexposed, as well as for those exposed to various levels of the factor, or to a combination of factors. The specific calculations of disease incidence in a given study will depend on whether the denominator includes numbers of individuals or person-time units of observation. Using these rates, both relative and absolute measures of association can be estimated and tested. The groups must also be compared to ensure similarity with respect to baseline differences that could be associated with the risk of developing the outcomes. Relative risk should be used in a cohort study to assess the likelihood of developing the disease in subjects who have been exposed to the risk factor, relative to those who have not been exposed. Attributable and population-attributable risks can also be calculated, and the Chi-squared test can be employed. However, one should be cautious when interpreting results, as a strong association does not necessarily indicate a causal relationship.

The longitudinal nature of cohort studies enables the assessment of causal hypotheses, as the exposure occurs prior to the outcome. Furthermore, measuring changes in levels of exposure over time alongside changes in outcome gives an insight into the dose-response relationship between exposure and outcome. Higher levels of exposure associated with higher levels of outcome provide further evidence for the causal relationship.

4. 3　Data Analysis

4.3.1　Measures of Outcome Frequency

4.3.1.1　Incidence Rate

The incidence rate is the rate at which new events occur in a population. The numerator is the number of new events that occur in a defined period or other physical spans. The denominator is the population at risk of experiencing the event during this period, sometimes expressed as person-time. The incidence rate most frequently used in public health practice is calculated from the following formula:

$$\text{Incidence rate} = \frac{\text{Number of new events in a specified period}}{\text{Average number of persons exposed to risk during this period}} \times 10^n$$

Strictly speaking, this ratio is neither a rate nor a proportion but is instead the rate multiplied by the length of the specified period. If the period is a year, the ratio is nonetheless often called the annual incidence rate. The average size of the population is often the estimated population size at the mid-period. The ratio divided by the length of the period is an estimate of the person-time incidence rate (e. g., the rate per 10^n person-years). If the ratio is small, as with many chronic diseases, it is also a good estimate of the cumulative incidence over the period (e. g., a year). If the number of new cases during a specified period is divided by the sum of the person-time units at risk for all persons during the period, the result is the person-time incidence rate.

4. 3. 1. 2   Cumulative Incidence (CI) (Synonym: Average Risk)

Cumulative incidence is the number or proportion of a group (cohort) of people who experience the onset of a health-related event during a specified time interval. This interval is generally the same for all members of the group, but, as in lifetime incidence, it may vary from person to person without reference to age. Cumulative incidence is simply defined as the ratio of incident cases to the population at risk at the beginning of the observation period. It describes a frequency measuring the proportion of individuals getting diseased.

$$CI = \frac{\text{Number of new cases of a specified outcome during a given period of time}}{\text{Total population at risk}}$$

The cumulative death rate is calculated in a similar way to specify the probability that an individual will die from a disease in a specified period. Cumulative incidence and death are often presented graphically so that the reader can see the estimated risk of an event for any duration of cohort follow-up. The cumulative probability of survival (or disease-free survival) is a comparable measure and represents the probability that an individual remains free of the outcome over the period of follow-up.

4. 3. 1. 3   Incidence Density (ID)

Incidence density is a summary estimate of the impact of exposure in a population that utilizes all available information over the entire period of follow-up. It represents the instantaneous rate of the occurrence of a specified outcome in a population and is defined as the following formula:

$$ID = \frac{\text{Number of new cases of a specified outcome during a given period of time}}{\text{Total person-time of observation}}$$

The numerator of the incidence density is the number of new cases in the population. The denominator is the sum of each individual's time at risk, or the sum of the time that each person remains under observation and free from the outcome.

4. 3. 1. 4   Standardized Mortality Ratio

The ratio of the number of deaths observed in the study group or population to the number that would be expected if the study population had the same specific rates as the standard population. It is often multiplied by 100.

In many retrospective cohort studies, such as those conducted in an occupational setting, the only available outcome information relates to the number of cases or deaths observed among the exposed cohort. The key research question is whether the number of cases in this group is unusual, that is, whether it is greater or less than one might have expected it to be. The standardized mortality ratio (SMR) and the standardized incidence ratio (SIR) may then be calculated. These measures represent the ratio of the observed number of deaths (or cases) among the study population divided by the expected number that would have occurred among the study population if it experiences the same pattern of mortality (or incidence) rates as the standard population.

4.3.2　Measures of Association

To facilitate a better understanding of measures of association between exposure and outcome, data from a cohort study can be conceptualized in the form of a two-by-two table shown in Table 4.1.

Table 4.1　Presentation of Data from a Cohort Study by a Two-by-Two Table

Exposure	Disease		Total
	Yes	No	
Yes	a	b	$a+b=n_1$
No	c	d	$c+d=n_0$
Total	$a+c=m_1$	$b+d=m_2$	$a+b+c+d=t$

Risk can be measured with relative risk, absolute risk or attributable risk.

4.3.2.1　Relative Risk (RR)

The RR is a ratio of the risk of an event among the exposed to the risk among the unexposed. This usage is synonymous with the risk ratio, but not synonymous with the odds ratio (OR). The use of OR to represent RR arises from the situation of "rare" (infrequent) diseases. For common occurrences, the approximations do not hold.

RR is defined as the ratio of the incidence of disease in the exposed group (expressed as I_1) divided by the corresponding incidence of disease in the unexposed group (I_0). Referring to table 4.1, the formula for calculating RR is:

$$RR = \frac{I_1}{I_0} = \frac{a/n_1}{c/n_0}$$

An RR of 1.0 indicates that the incidence rates of disease in the exposed and unexposed groups are identical and that there is no association between the exposure and outcome. A value greater than 1.0 indicates a positive association or an increased risk among those exposed to the factor. Analogously, a RR of less than 1.0 means that there is an inverse association or a decreased risk among exposed groups.

The confidence interval that surrounds an estimate of the RR can be calculated using the following formula:

$$95\%CI = (RR)\exp(1.96\sqrt{Var(\ln RR)})$$

$$Var(\ln RR) = \frac{1}{a} + \frac{1}{b} + \frac{1}{c} + \frac{1}{d}$$

4.3.2.2　Attributable Risk (AR) (Synonym: Risk Difference)

AR is the proportion of the rate (risk) of a disease or other outcome in exposed individuals that can be attributed to the exposure. It is defined as the difference between the incidence rates in the exposed and unexposed groups and can be calculated as the following formula:

$$AR = I_1 - I_0 = I_0(RR - 1)$$

The AR is used to quantify the amount of disease risk that can be considered to be a result of the exposure in the exposed group after removing the risk of disease that would have occurred anyway due to other causes (the risk in the unexposed). It indicates the incidence rate of the disease among the exposed that can be attributed to the exposure itself, or alternatively, the incidence among the exposed that could theoretically be avoided if the exposure were eliminated.

It is important to remember that RR and AR provide different information on the association between the exposure and outcome. The RR is a measure of the strength of the association between exposure and disease, which can be used to judge the causal relationship. In contrast, the AR provides a measure of the possible public health impact of the presumed cause.

In general, the RR is the measure used most commonly by those evaluating possible determinants of disease, since it represents the magnitude of the association and can be used in making a judgment of causality. From the perspective of public health administration and policy, in contrast, once causality is assumed, measures of association based on absolute differences in risk between exposed and unexposed individuals assume far greater importance. These absolute rates express either the actual incidence of a disease that is attributable to exposure among the exposed (AR) or the incidence of disease in the total population that could be eliminated by removal of a harmful exposure (population attributable risk).

4.3.2.3　Attributable Risk Percent (AR%) (Synonym: Etiologic Fraction)

To estimate the proportion of a disease among the exposed that is attributable to the exposure or the proportion of a disease in a group that might be prevented by eliminating the exposure, one may use the attributable risk percent (AR%).

$$AR\% = \frac{(I_1 - I_0)}{I_1} \times 100\% = \frac{RR - 1}{RR} \times 100\%$$

4.3.2.4　Population Attributable Risk (PAR)

The PAR can be used to estimate the excess incidence rate of the disease that is attributable to the exposure in the total cohort. It provides insights into which exposures have the most relevance to the health of a community. The PAR is calculated as the incidence rate of disease in the population (I_t) minus the incidence rate in the unexposed group (I_0).

$$PAR = I_t - I_0$$

The AR among the exposed will always be greater than the PAR since the impact of removing the exposure on disease incidence will always be greater for those with the exposure than for a total population, which is a combination of exposed and unexposed individuals.

4.3.2.5　Population Attributable Risk Percent (PAR%)

This is the attributable fraction in the population expressed as a percentage. PAR% is calculated using the following formula:

$$PAR\% = \frac{I_t - I_0}{I_t} \times 100\% = \frac{Pe(RR - 1)}{Pe(RR - 1) + 1} \times 100\%$$

4.3.3 Survival Analysis

For certain outcomes (e. g. , mortality and renal allograft failure), it may be particularly relevant to consider the time until the event occurs, rather than the incidence of the event. For example, the incidence of death would be equal in all subgroups of a cohort if they are followed for a long period of time, regardless of any true association between exposure and risk. However, even when the outcome is not inevitable, refining estimates of risk by considering the time to the event usually results in increased statistical power compared with analyses that simply evaluate whether the event occurred. Two commonly used techniques include Kaplan-Meier analysis and Cox proportional hazards analysis.

4.3.4 Reporting Cohort Studies

Many researchers report their findings of cohort studies in an unsatisfactory way. An investigator's first challenge is to convince the editor (then readers) that the exposed and unexposed groups were indeed similar in all important aspects, except for the exposure. The first table in reporting cohort studies customarily provides demographic and other prognostic factors for both groups with hypothesis testing (p values) to show the likelihood that the observed differences could be due to chance. For dichotomous outcome measures, such as sick or well, the investigator should provide sufficient raw data for the reader. For cumulative incidence, the investigator should calculate the proportion that developed the outcome during the specified study interval. For the incidence rate, the value is expressed per unit of time. Then, RR with 95% CI should be provided. Like other observational studies, cohort studies have a built-in bias. Investigators should identify potential biases and show how these might have affected the results. Whenever possible, confounding should be controlled in the analysis. Important features needed to be checked in a cohort study are listed in Table 4. 2.

Table 4. 2 Features to Look for in a Cohort Study

Questions

1. How much selection bias was present?
- Were only people at risk of the outcome included?
- Was the exposure clear, specific, and measurable?
- Were the exposed and unexposed groups similar in all important respects except for the exposure?

2. What steps were taken to minimize information bias?
- Was the outcome clear, specific, and measurable?
- Was the outcome identified in the same way for both groups?
- Was determination of outcome made by an observer blinded as to treatment?

3. How complete was the follow-up of both groups?
- What efforts were made to limit loss to follow-up?
- Was loss to follow-up similar in both groups?

(To be continued)

Table 4. 2

Questions
4. Were potential confounding factors sought and controlled for in the analysis?   • Did the investigators anticipate and gather information on potential confounding factors?   • What methods were used to assess and control for confounding?

In order to improve the inadequate reporting of observational studies, the initiative named Strengthening the Reporting of Observational Studies in Epidemiology (STROBE) developed a 22-item checklist, with recommendations about what should be included in a more accurate and complete description of observational studies (Table 4. 3).

Table 4. 3   The STROBE Statement—Checklist of Items that Should Be Included in Reports of Cohort Studies

Item	No.	Recommendation
Title and abstract	1	(a) Indicate the study's design with a commonly used term in the title or the abstract
		(b) Provide in the abstract an informative and balanced summary of what was done and what was found
Introduction		
Background/ rationale	2	Explain the scientific background and rationale for the investigation being reported
Objectives	3	State specific objectives, including any prespecified hypotheses
Methods		
Study design	4	Present key elements of study design early in the paper
Setting	5	Describe the setting, locations, and relevant dates, including periods of recruitment, exposure, follow-up, and data collection
Participants	6	(a) Give the eligibility criteria and the sources and methods of selection of participants. Describe methods of follow-up
		(b) For matched studies, give matching criteria and number of exposed and unexposed
Variables	7	Clearly define all outcomes, exposures, predictors, potential confounders, and effect modifiers. Give diagnostic criteria, if applicable
Data sources/ measurement	8*	For each variable of interest, give sources of data and details of methods of assessment (measurement). Describe comparability of assessment methods if there is more than one group
Bias	9	Describe any efforts to address potential sources of bias
Study size	10	Explain how the study size was arrived at
Quantitative variables	11	Explain how quantitative variables were handled in the analyses. If applicable, describe which groupings were chosen and why

(To be continued)

Table 4. 3

Item	No.	Recommendation
Statistical methods	12	(a) Describe all statistical methods, including those used to control for confounding
		(b) Describe any methods used to examine subgroups and interactions
		(c) Explain how missing data were addressed
		(d) If applicable, explain how the loss to follow-up was addressed
		(e) Describe any sensitivity analyses

Results

Item	No.	Recommendation
Participants	13*	(a) Report numbers of individuals at each stage of study—e. g. , numbers potentially eligible, examined for eligibility, confirmed eligible, included in the study, completing follow-up, and analyzed
		(b) Give reasons for non-participation at each stage
		(c) Consider use of a flow diagram
Descriptive data	14*	(a) Give characteristics of study participants (e. g. , demographic, clinical, social) and information on exposures and potential confounders
		(b) Indicate number of participants with missing data for each variable of interest
		(c) Summarize follow-up time (e. g. , average and total amount)
Outcome data	15*	Report numbers of outcome events or summary measures over time
Main results	16	(a) Give unadjusted estimates and, if applicable, confounder-adjusted estimates and their precision (e. g. , 95% confidence interval). Make clear which confounders were adjusted for and why they were included
		(b) Report category boundaries when continuous variables were categorized
		(c) If relevant, consider translating estimates of relative risk into absolute risk for a meaningful time period
Other analyses	17	Report other analyses done—e. g. , analyses of subgroups and interactions, and sensitivity analyses

Discussion

Item	No.	Recommendation
Key results	18	Summarize key results with reference to study objectives
Limitations	19	Discuss limitations of the study, taking into account sources of potential bias or imprecision. Discuss both direction and magnitude of any potential bias
Interpretation	20	Give a cautious overall interpretation of results considering objectives, limitations, multiplicity of analyses, results from similar studies, and other relevant evidence
Generalizability	21	Discuss the generalizability (external validity) of the study results

Other Information

Item	No.	Recommendation
Funding	22	Give the source of funding and the role of the funders for the present study and, if applicable, for the original study on which the present article is based

* Give information separately for exposed and unexposed groups.

Note: Information on the STROBE Initiative is available at http://www. strobe-statement. org.

4. 4   Bias

Observational studies, compared with randomized controlled trials, often include participants with a broader spectrum of disease severity and comorbidity. Therefore, results from
cohort studies highlighting the effects of treatment may have better generalizability to the
affected population than those from randomized trials. However, risks for drawing incorrect
inferences about treatment effects from cohort studies tend to be higher because of the increased likelihood of bias; therefore, randomized trials should be applied to confirm the results from observational studies whenever possible.

Bias is a systematic deviation of results or inferences from the truth. This is an error
that may occur in the conception and design of a study, or in the recruitment of participants,
in data collection, analysis, interpretation, reporting, or publication, leading to results or
conclusions that are systematically (as opposed to randomly) different from the truth. Although a number of potential biases may occur, three major categories are commonly used:
selection bias, information bias, and confounding.

4. 4. 1   Selection Bias

Selection bias may also appear in cohort studies in case that the exposed and unexposed
groups are not truly comparable. One example is the length-time bias, which occurs when
participants with a moderate disease are preferentially enrolled because they are more likely
to follow the course allowing a longer period for detection and a higher likelihood of participating. This is because pathophysiology, natural history, and expected response to treatment may differ substantially in those with moderate as compared to severe forms of the disease. Selection bias may also be introduced due to the loss of follow up, thus maintaining a
high level of follow up among all study groups can minimize this type of bias.

4. 4. 1. 1   The Effects of Nonparticipation

In reality, only a proportion of those who are eligible to participate actually agree to do
so and are enrolled in the study. Volunteers participating in a cohort study may differ from
individuals who do not participate in various characteristics such as age, gender, race, economic status, or education level. A positive finding in a sampled study population does not
eliminate the possibility that such a bias does not exist, or that it exists to a different degree, among persons not included in the cohort.

4. 4. 1. 2   Loss to Follow-up Bias

A major source of potential section bias in cohort studies is the loss to follow-up. Cohort participants may migrate, change jobs, die or just refuse to continuously participate in
the study. The loss to follow-up may be related to the exposure, outcome or both. For example, individuals who develop the outcome may be less likely to continue to be followed up

in the study. Therefore, loss to follow-up bias represents a threat to the internal validity of estimates derived from cohort studies.

4.4.1.3 Healthy Worker Effect

Healthy worker effect is another potential form of selection bias in cohort studies, particularly affecting occupational studies. In an occupational cohort study where disease rates among individuals from a particular occupational group are compared with an external standard population, bias may be introduced if membership of the exposed cohort is partly dependent upon health. Individuals who are employed, for example, are generally healthy by nature of their ability to work. Mortality or morbidity rate in this group may be initially lower than that in the general population. To minimize this type of bias, a comparison group may be selected from a group of workers with different jobs performed at different locations within a single facility. Alternatively, the comparison group may be selected from an external population of employed individuals.

4.4.2　Information Bias

Information bias can be introduced when information of exposure or outcome is systematically incorrect, either when the exposure is measured differently in people with the outcome or when the likelihood of detecting the outcome varies between exposed and unexposed persons. Conversely, misclassification of exposure or outcome that occurs at random (non-differential misclassification) will tend to bias toward the null value (the finding that exposure and outcome are not associated). The effect of random misclassification, in general, is to obscure the distinction between the exposed and unexposed groups so that any true association between the exposure and outcome will be distorted. Differential misclassification, on the other hand, occurs when the errors in the classification of individuals by exposure or disease produce a differential accuracy or quality of information among the study groups. The effect is either underestimated or overestimated or by chance, the same as the true measure of association.

Although statistical techniques can be used to compensate partially some types of bias, it's better to prevent them by appropriate study design. In case the study design cannot be changed, sensitivity analyses can provide reassurance about the potential impact of these biases.

4.4.3　Confounding Bias

Confounding is the bias of the estimated effect of an exposure on an outcome due to the presence of a common cause of the exposure and the outcome. A classic example of confounding is the observation that coffee drinkers are at higher risk for lung cancer. In this example, cigarette smoking is a confounder, because it is associated with both the exposure (smokers are more likely to drink coffee) and the outcome (smoking is a risk factor of lung cancer).

A confounder is a factor that must be associated with both the exposure, independent of that exposure and the outcome. Moreover, confounders should not be involved directly in the causal pathway between exposure and outcome. For example, in studies of the relation between smoking and CVD risk, increased blood pressure might be associated with both the exposure (smoking) and the outcome (CVD), but may not confound the association because increased blood pressure may be involved in the causal pathway between smoking and CVD.

In assessing the effect of a potential confounder, it is important to evaluate its presence or absence and the direction (positive or negative) and magnitude of its effect on the estimate of the association between the risk factor and the disease. Several methods can be employed, independently or in combination, to control for confounding in cohort studies. During the study design phase, matching and restriction may be used, and during the data analysis phase, the statistical techniques such as stratification and multivariate regression can be used.

4.5   Strengths and Limitations

4.5.1   Strengths of Cohort Studies

①It can measure the incidence and prevalence rate of a disease.

②It can calculate RR.

③It shows a clear temporal relationship between exposure and disease, demonstrating the direction of causality.

④It can be used to measure the effect of rare exposures.

⑤It can yield information on multiple outcomes due to a particular exposure.

⑥It has less bias.

⑦It provides strong evidence for establishing cause and effect relationship.

4.5.2   Limitations of Cohort Studies

①It is costly and time-consuming.

②It often requires a large sample size.

③There are poor choices for the study on rare diseases.

④It is prone to bias due to loss to follow-up.

⑤Classification of individuals (exposure or outcome status) can be affected by changes in diagnostic procedures.

⑥Knowledge of exposure status may bias the classification of the outcome.

⑦Being recruited in the study may alter the participant's behavior.

4.5.3   Ethical Consideration

It is now generally accepted that studies on humans should be carried out with informed consent. This principle, originally developed in relation to controlled clinical trials, has been extended to observational epidemiology studies, including cohort studies. Currently, many cohorts need to collect biological specimens (e. g. , blood, buccal cells, DNA), and in this case, it becomes mandatory that consent for the future use of such specimens for research purposes should be provided by the respondent. However, at the time the specimens are requested, it is impossible to know exactly the precise use the investigators may wish to apply to this material. An example is the cohort study of the European Prospective Investigation of Diet and Cancer (Riboli and Kaaks, 1997). Participants provided blood specimens in the early 1990s. The majority signed a consent form. However, now that genetic studies are commonplace on such specimens, it has become apparent that previously signed consent forms did not specifically mention genetic analyses as potential research usages. This has led to difficulties in obtaining approval for such studies from human experimentation committees, some of which wanted new consent forms to be signed, specific to the genetically-associated sub-study planned. Obtaining new consent, however, will become increasingly difficult as time goes on, and a number of subjects with the endpoint of interest may have died. In Europe, there has been a more relaxed view of the ethical acceptability of studies on stored specimens, many such collections having been originally made without a formal informed consent process, but for which studies conducted with full preservation of confidentiality have been deemed to be ethically acceptable. The issue as to whether respondents whose stored specimens have been tested should be informed of the results of such tests is also controversial. The European view tends to be that as the testing is being conducted as part of the research, it may be impossible to interpret the results of tests for individuals until this particular research track reaches agreed conclusions. Thus, it is not necessary, indeed possibly unethical, to inform the respondent of the results. In the United States, however, the opposite viewpoint says that it is regarded as ethically inappropriate for investigators to take a decision on whether or not a subject receives information on themselves. The difficulty with a universal application of such a principle is that for some, the test results may come too late for any possibility of benefit, but, especially in the case of genetically-related information, this may not preclude the test result having implications for the relatives of the subject, and such knowledge is not always a blessing. However, all would agree that if a test reveals information of potential benefit to a subject, they should be informed.

The question of consent for historical cohort studies, in general, does not arise, though again, there may be issues on informing subjects of the findings of the research. In general, as the research is unlikely to harm the individuals, and providing confidentiality is maintained, human experimentation committees will approve such studies.

4. 6 Summary

Cohort studies, in particular, prospective cohort studies, offer several important advantages compared to other forms of observational studies. A cohort study is a critical method for evaluating causality in epidemiology, and is often ranked at a higher level of evidence than a case-control study, largely because the latter is susceptible to recall bias. However, both case-control studies and cohorts are usually regarded as "level Ⅱ" evidence (level Ⅰ are randomized controlled trials). There are potential deficiencies in cohort studies that may be less intrusive than in case-control studies, especially a greater propensity for measurement error. It is certain that the evidence for any link between exposure and outcome rarely relies on a single study, regardless of the study design, and requires aggregate support from a multitude of biologic, translational, and clinical studies.

(Lu Guangyu, Wang Jianming)

Exercise

Chapter 5   Case-Control Study

5.1   Introduction

Case-control study is one of the most important methodology of modern epidemiology. Conceptually, there are clear links from randomized experiments to nonrandomized cohort studies, and from nonrandomized cohort studies to case-control studies. Case-control studies nevertheless differ from the scientific paradigm of experimentation. There is a long history for the case-control study design, extending back at least to Guy's 1843 comparison of the occupations of men with pulmonary consumption to the occupations of men having other diseases. Beginning in the 1920s, it was used to link cancer to environmental and hormonal exposures. The landmark study of Doll and Hill (1950, 1952), in particular, inspired future generations of epidemiologists to use this methodology. It remains to this day a model for the design and conduct of case-control studies, with excellent suggestions on how to reduce or eliminate selection, interview and recall bias. In this chapter, we will introduce the definition and designs of a case-control study, explain how to conduct a case-control study, and discuss its advantages and disadvantages, mainly compared with a cohort design. We also consider variants of the basic case-control study design.

5.1.1   Definition of Case-Control Study

Case-control study is an analytic epidemiologic research design in which the study population consists of groups who either have (cases) or do not have (controls) a particular health problem or outcome. The investigator looks back in time to measure the exposure of the study subjects. The exposure is then compared between cases and controls to determine if the exposure could account for the health condition of the cases. For example, if we want to assess the association between smoking and lung cancer using a case-control study design, first we should select a group of patients who have already suffered lung cancer as cases, and then we should select another group of participants without lung cancer as controls. Subsequently, smoking information was collected by questionnaires. If the proportion of smokers in the case group is significantly higher than those in the control group, this indicates that smoking might be associated with risk of lung cancer. But we need to be aware that this association may not be a causal one. Even excluding random errors and known systematic errors, the association between exposure and disease may be also affected by unknown factors.

5. 1. 2　Basic Principals of Case-Control Study

A case-control study is designed to help determine if an exposure is associated with an outcome (i. e. , disease or condition of interest). Case-control studies can be described in a simple way. First, we identify the cases (a group known to have the outcome) and the controls (a group known to be free of the outcome). Then, we retrospectively investigate which subjects in each group had the exposure(s) and compare the frequency of the exposure between case group and control group. Information may be collected for both cases and controls on genetic, social, behavioral, environmental or other determinants of the disease.

The primary feature that distinguishes a case-control study from a cohort study is the selection of subjects based on their disease status. The investigator selects cases from those persons who have the disease of interest and controls from those who do not. In a well-designed case-control study, cases are selected from a clearly defined population, sometimes called the source population, and controls are selected from the same population that yield the cases. The prior exposure for both cases and controls are examined to assess the relationship between exposure and disease. The basic design of a case-control study is shown in Figure 5. 1.

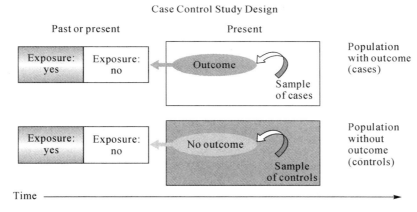

Figure 5. 1　Schematic Diagram of Case-Control Study Design (Schulz KF and Grimes DA, 2002)

The aspects of comparability that must be considered include factors such as the baseline risk of developing the disease other than from the exposure(s) under study, as well as the accuracy and completeness of data. Consequently, the major issues to be considered in designing and conducting a case-control study are the selection of the study groups and the sources of information about exposure and disease.

By definition, a case-control study is always retrospective because it starts with an outcome then traces back to investigate exposures. When the subjects are enrolled in their respective groups, the outcome of each subject is already known by the investigator. This, and not the fact that the investigator usually makes use of previously collected data, is what makes case-control studies "retrospective".

Well designed case-control studies can provide valuable information for the association between exposure and disease. In fact, because of their advantage in being able to evaluate diseases that have already occurred for many years following relevant exposures in a timely and cost-effective manner, case-control studies have become the most common analytic epidemiologic study design encountered in the medical literature today.

5.1.3 Types of Case-Control Study

Confounding is a distortion of results that occurs when the apparent effects of the exposure of interest are attributable entirely or in part to the effects of an extraneous variable. Confounding is likely to occur when persons exposed to the risk factor of interest differ from non-exposed persons with respect to the prevalence of other risk factors for the disease of interest. Matching is a popular approach to control confounding in case-control studies. According to matching status, a case-control study design can be either matched or non-matched.

For the non-matched case-control study, control are selected from a population without being specifically matched to cases. Instead, the matched case-control study design forces the case group and the control group to be similar with respect to important risk factors and thereby makes case-control comparisons less subject to confounding. The first step in matching is to identify a case. Investigators then select from the source population one or more potential controls who have the same values that the case has for each matching factor. To match on a continuous variable such as age, it is typically necessary to form categories, such as 5-year intervals (10 — 14, 15 — 19, 20 — 24 years, etc.). In a study with matching on race, sex, and age in 5-year intervals, a 17-year-old African-American female case would be matched to an African-American female control aged 15 — 19 from the source population. As in an unmatched study, these controls would come from the defined source population. More than one control can be matched to each case, but the ratio of controls to cases rarely exceeds 4 : 1 because additional controls beyond this ratio add relatively little to the statistical power of the study.

Matching is commonly used in case-control studies on rare diseases. In this situation, there are a small number of potential cases and a large number of potential controls. Matching can increase the statistical efficiency, thus achieving a particular level of statistical power with a small sample size. The matching protocol often simplifies decisions about how to select controls. In addition, matching tends to ensure that differences in the risk factor of interest cannot be explained by reference to the matching variables.

However, these advantages of matching must be weighed against a number of disadvantages. As indicated above, matching can be time-consuming and therefore expensive. Any potential cases or controls that cannot be matched must be discarded, which can be viewed as a wasteful process. Any variable that is matched in a study cannot be evaluated as a risk factor in that investigation. And matching on ordinal or continuous variables may result in categories that are too broad to remove the effects of the matched variables completely from the exposure-disease relationship. Table 5.1 shows the advantages and disadvantages of matching in case-control studies.

Table 5.1   **Advantages and Disadvantages of Matching in Case-Control Studies**

Advantages	Disadvantages
May increase the precision of case-control comparisons and thus allow a smaller sample size	May be time-consuming and expensive to perform
The sampling process is easy to understand and explain	Some potential cases and controls may be excluded because matches cannot be made
If analyzed correctly, it provides reassurance that matched variables cannot explain case-control differences in the risk factor of interest	The matched variables cannot be evaluated as risk factors in the study population
	For continuous or ordinal variables, matching categories may be too broad, and residual case-control differences in these variables may persist

Overmatching refers to matching on a factor that is not a confounder, for example, the factor related only to exposure, the factor related only to disease, or the factor that is an intermediate in the exposure-disease causal pathway.

5.1.4   Application of Case-Control Studies

Case-Control studies are increasingly used to explore the causes of a disease and other important health events, particularly suitable for exploring the causes of unexplained diseases. The case-control study is also useful for exploring factors that are predictors of a drug's curative effects and side effects. Treatments can have both beneficial and adverse outcomes, so identifying factors associated with these outcomes is a crucial aspect in clinical researches. Another important advantage of case-control studies is that they provide an efficient way of exploring prognostic factors of disease. "Prognosis" refers to the future course of the disease (including death, complications, disability, etc.) and the results of case-control studies that identify prognostic factors may lead to interventions that improve patient's outcomes.

5.2   Design and Implementation of Case-Control Studies

For a case-control study to provide sound evidence of whether there is a valid statistical association between exposure and disease, the ability to compare cases and controls is essential. One of the first steps in a case-control study is to identify and select cases—a step that also determines the source population. Another important step in designing a case-control study is to specify the definition of a case. The next key step in a case-control study is to identify and select controls. Ideally, controls are chosen randomly from the source population. Once cases and controls are selected, the next step is to obtain information as accurate as possible about each individual's prior exposure to the risk factor of interest.

5.2.1 Selection of Cases

Case should be well defined. For example, cases might be sampled randomly from all patients who are diagnosed during the study period and who reside within a certain geographic region. These cases may be identified by a surveillance system or by interviewing hospital records, other medical records, or death certificates available through institutional or population-based disease registries. In some situations, complete identification of cases in a well-defined source population may be too time-consuming or otherwise infeasible. If so, a common alternative involves the use of a "convenience sample". Cases might be sampled from patients admitted to particular hospitals or from those seen in certain clinics. Although such cases can often be identified easily, the underlying source population may not be well defined, thus making it difficult to generalize results.

5.2.1.1 Types of Cases

The investigator typically studies newly diagnosed or incident cases, although it is sometimes necessary to include previously existing or prevalent cases. Prevalent cases should be avoided if the exposure has the potential to affect the prognosis or the duration of the illness. When this effect occurs, the exposure status of existing prevalent cases tends to differ from that of all cases. The general principle is that the likelihood of a case being included in the study must not depend on the exposure.

5.2.1.2 Sources of Cases

(1) Population Registries

Population-based disease registries, particularly for cancer and birth defects, are often considered the ideal source of cases. Practical limitations on their use include the time-consuming of case identification and investigation, and selection bias due to the exclusion of those who may have died, and the feasibility of random sampling of controls.

(2) Hospitals and Clinics

Historically, many case-control studies have been conducted in a single or a small group of hospitals or clinics. This facilitates timely access to cases and increases the likelihood of their cooperation, thus limiting selection bias. On the other hand, the definition of the source population from which the cases arise may be problematic, not to mention the practicality of obtaining random samples of controls from it.

(3) Health Maintenance Organizations

Large health maintenance organizations (HMOs) are also considered as a source of cases. The source population is enumerated and demographic data, as well as some exposure and covariate data, may already be available for everyone. This permits judicious selection of cases and controls using the nested case-control, case-cohort or stratified two-phase sampling designs. Relatively objective and inexpensive exposure assessments may be possible using routine medical or pharmacy records, some of which may already exist in the electronic form. Similarly, cases are usually easily ascertained from reports of diagnoses within the organization. Of course, some assurance are needed that the members of HMO are unlikely to go elsewhere for diagnosis and treatment.

5. 2. 2　Selection of Controls

Ideally, controls are chosen randomly from the source population. If the source population is a state, city, or other well-defined areas, controls can be contacted by dialing telephone numbers randomly (random-digit dialing), by visiting residences, by mailing letters soliciting participation, or by other means. An important goal is to select controls without depending on exposure. That is to say, the sample of controls should have the same prevalence of exposure as the source population of unaffected persons. If the selection of controls is related to the exposure, the case-control comparison may be distorted.

5. 2. 2. 1　Principles of Control Selection

Wacholder et al. described three basic principles of control selection. The first two correspond roughly to considerations already developed regarding conceptual foundations and the use of matching. The third one stems from the desire to minimize the effects of measurement error to which case-control studies are particularly susceptible. In view of the drawbacks of overmatching, and the modest efficiency gains even when statistical adjustment is indicated, one may well ask whether matching is ever justified. The administrative costs of locating matched controls, and the loss of cases from analysis if none can be found, further argue for careful consideration of matched designs. Individual case-control matching is mostly appealing when you want to control the effects of a confounder that is not easily measured. Greater attention to the stratification of the control sample may be needed when the primary goal is to evaluate statistical interaction, or effect modification, between the exposure and covariate.

(1) The "Study-Base" Principle

This is the principle that controls should be randomly selected from disease-free members of an underlying cohort, also known as the source population or study-base, at the times that cases are being ascertained. When controls are selected later, it sometimes mandates the random selection of a reference date for each control so that the diagnosis dates for cases and reference dates for controls are comparable. Only exposures occurring prior to the reference date of diagnosis would be considered.

(2) The Deconfounding Principle

This principle underlies the stratified sampling of controls to render possibility, or improve the efficiency of, an adjusted analysis designed to control confounding.

(3) The Comparable Accuracy Principle

This principle suggests that the measurement error of exposures and covariates among controls is comparable to that among cases. For example, the suggestion that dead controls should be selected for dead cases, is sometimes made on the basis of the comparable accuracy principle. Unfortunately, there is no guarantee that adherence to the principle will eliminate or even reduce bias. Unless the measurement error can be completely controlled, it can seriously compromise the validity of the study even if the case and control data are equally error-prone.

5. 2. 2. 2   Sources of Controls

The appropriate source population for the sampling of controls is determined by the study-base principal. When cases arise from an enumerated source population such as the HMO, controls may be sampled from this cohort using a nested case-control or case-cohort design. Standard survey sampling methods are often used to select controls for "population-based" studies in countries that do not maintain population registers. The most difficult and controversial problems on control selection arise with hospital-based studies.

(1) Hospital-Based Controls

Many studies that ascertain cases through hospitals also select controls from the same hospitals, which is of obvious logistical convenience. Such controls are likely to have the same high response levels as the cases. The fact that they may be interviewed in a hospital setting, as the cases are, is an advantage from the perspective of the comparable accuracy principle. The major difficulties stem from the fact that the hypothetical study-base, and the catchment of persons who would report to the particular hospital if they develop the disease under study, may be different from the catchment population for other diseases. Furthermore, many of the disease categories from which controls could be selected may be associated with the exposure. A large part of the planning of hospital-based case-control studies is devoted to the choice of disease categories thought to be independent of exposure and to have a similar catchment. The hope is that controls with such diseases will effectively constitute a random sample from the study-base. Since the independence of exposure and disease diagnosis is rarely known with great certainty, a standard recommendation is to select controls having a variety of diagnoses so that the failure of any one of them to meet the criterion does not compromise the study. If it is found later that a certain diagnosis is associated with exposure, those controls can be excluded.

(2) Neighborhood and Friend Controls

Matched controls may also be selected from neighbors or friends of cases. For the former method, a census is taken of all households in the immediate geographic area of the case and these are approached in a random order until a suitable control is found. Care must be taken to ensure that the control is the resident at the same time when the case is diagnozed. Even with these precautions, neighborhood sampling may yield biased controls for hospital-based studies since it will not be guaranteed that the control would have been ascertained when the case is diagnozed, thus violating the study-base principle. Neighborhood controls are also susceptible to overmatching due to their similarity to the cases on factors associated with the exposure that are not risk factors. The same difficulties confront the use of friend controls, whereby a random selection is taken from a census of friends provided by each case. There may be further selection on factors related to popularity since the friend being selected as the control may have not listed the case as a friend. The primary advantage of friend controls would be a low level of nonresponse.

(3) Survey Sampling

Methods for scientific sampling of populations have been developed by census bureaus and other government agencies throughout the world. The particular method most advantageous for any given epidemiologic study will likely depend on the local administrative infrastructure. Survey sampling often proceeds in stages, by firstly sampling a large administrative unit, then selecting a smaller one and finally arriving at an individual household or subject. Such multi-stage "cluster" sampling introduces modest correlations in the response of individuals sampled from the same primary sampling unit, more marked ones for individuals sampled from the same lower level cluster. Although often ignored by epidemiologists, these correlations should be accounted for in the rigorous statistical analysis. Fortunately, simple methods to accommodate cluster sampling are now routinely incorporated in the standard statistical packages.

(4) Random Digit Dialing

In view of the high costs of census bureau techniques in the United States, methods of survey sampling through the telephone exchanges have been developed. Random digit dialing (RDD) has become increasingly popular for control selection in populations that have high rates of telephone access. Some implementations start with the telephone exchange of each case for the sampling of controls that are thereby matched on somewhat ill-defined neighborhood factors. RDD methods may be costly for the ascertainment of controls from minority populations, requiring dozens of calls to locate a suitable household. They are particularly susceptible to bias because of higher selection probabilities for households that have more than one phone line or more than one eligible control and because of high rates of nonresponse. The latter problem is likely to become increasingly serious in view of the persistent use of answering machines to screen out unwanted calls. The popularity of cell phones, moreover, eventually may make it infeasible to use RDD to draw a random control sample from a source population defined by geographic or administrative boundaries.

5.2.3   Sample Size Estimation

In calculating the required sample size for a case-control study, it is necessary to specify the desired values for the probabilities of type I (alpha) and type II (beta) errors, and for the proportion of the baseline population that is exposed to the factor of interest and the expected magnitude of the effect. Once these values have been specified, the necessary sample size can be determined using one of a number of standard formulas.

The sample size determined using a formula should be interpreted as providing a minimum estimate of the desired sample sizes for the study because this formula takes into account only the estimate of the overall crude association between exposure and disease. It does not consider the statistical consequences of control of potential confounding factors. Also, if the investigators expect to conduct analyses confined to subgroups of the study population, larger numbers will be required to have adequate statistical power.

Supposed the ratio of the number of cases relative to that of controls was $1 : c$, the following formula(5. 1) is used to estimate sample size for an unmatched case-control study:

$$n= \left(1+\frac{1}{c}\right) \times \bar{p} \times \bar{q} \times \frac{(z_\alpha + z_\beta)^2}{(p_1 - p_0)^2} \tag{5. 1}$$

$$\bar{p} = 0.5 \times (p_1 + p_0) \tag{5. 2}$$

$$\bar{q} = 1 - \bar{p} \tag{5. 3}$$

p_1—the frequency of exposure among cases; p_0—the frequency of exposure among controls (baseline population); Z_α—the standard normal deviation based on different desired values of α; Z_β—the standard normal deviation based on different desired values of β.

5. 2. 4　Measurements of Exposure and Disease Status

5. 2. 4. 1　Measurements of Exposure

The information about each individual's prior exposure to the risk factor of interest, as well as to other exposures, should be collected as accurate as possible. The information concerning other exposures is used to determine whether the association of the disease with a factor is due to the exposure of interest or to other characteristics of exposed persons. Because factors cannot affect risk after the disease occurs, the timing of exposures is critical. For chronic diseases that lack early evidence of involvement, establishing the temporal sequence of exposure and onset of disease can be difficult or impossible.

5. 2. 4. 2　Measurements of Disease Status

The definition of a case should be specified. The criteria should minimize the likelihood that an affected person (true case) is missed (i. e. , the criteria must be sensitive) or that a non-affected person is falsely classified as a case (i. e. , the criteria must be specific). In general, there is a trade-off between the desire to include all cases and the desire to prevent dilution of the case group with non-affected persons. Moreover, restrictive criteria may require information that is unavailable for some subjects, making it impossible for such subjects to be classified fully. In practice, inclusion criteria are chosen to minimize misclassification yet to promote feasibility.

5. 2. 5　Data Collection

Information concerning risk factors may be obtained from medical, occupational, or other records. These methods of obtaining information are not based on self-reporting and can avoid the reporting bias. The amount of information found in records is often limited. Furthermore, this information may not be recorded in a standardized manner, leading to variability in subject classification.

Interviews and questionnaires are the most common means of determining a subject's exposure history. Interviews can be conducted face to face or by telephone. To ensure that information from cases and controls is obtained in the same manner, interviews should be standardized, monitored, and conducted by trained interviewers. Interviews are useful for collecting data because ①questions may cover a wide range of potential risk factors, ②costs are relatively low, and ③information of exposures that occurred years prior to the onset of illness can be obtained. Occasionally, there is a concern that cases and controls may recall exposures differently, perhaps distorting case-control comparison. For example, cases—perhaps in an attempt to explain their illnesses—may over-report exposures. This is of particular concern when there has been a great deal of publicity about the association between the exposure and the disease of interest. For instance, after the association of smoking with lung cancer was first identified and publicized, knowledge of this association could have affected the reported exposures of cases in subsequent investigations.

The most objective means of characterizing exposure is through the use of a biological marker in blood or other specimens. There are several difficulties inherent in the use of biological markers, however. First, obtaining the specimens can involve an invasive procedure that discourages subject participation. Second, many diseases do not have known biological markers. Third, even if a marker exists, it may be transient and thus not present when the measurement is taken. Finally, the disease state may alter metabolism, thereby distorting case-control comparisons.

5.3   Data Analysis of Case-Control Study

5.3.1   Descriptive Analysis

After the information is collected, the data should be cleaned immediately. This is mainly a process that involves identifying missing data items, ensuring that coded responses are within a reasonable range, checking for logical inconsistencies between different data fields, and deleting data for subjects who are ineligible for the study. Once the data is clean, the general characteristics (e. g. , age, gender, occupation, etc.) of case and control groups should be compared directly to assess possible differences in factors that could be associated with the risk of developing the outcome under study.

5.3.2   Statistical Inference

The statistical inference employed in a case-control study depends on whether subjects were sampled in an unmatched or in a matched approach. These two analytic strategies are described in the following sections.

5.3.2.1 Unmatched Design

The data obtained in an unmatched case-control study can be summarized as indicated in table 5.2. For simplicity, only two levels of exposure are discussed here, although the basic methods can be expanded to include multiple levels of exposure. Each subject can be classified into one of four basic groups defined by disease and prior exposure status.

Although the summary tables for cohort and case-control studies appear similar, it is important to remember that the underlying approaches to sampling differ, and the analysis must account for these differences. In a cohort study, sampling is based on exposure status, and the investigator thus determines the totals numbers of exposed $(a+b)$ and unexposed subjects $(c+d)$ in the study. Then the risk of disease development can be estimated separately for exposed and unexposed groups, and compared in a risk ratio (RR) or relative risk (RR).

Table 5.2　Summary of Data Collected in an Unmatched Case-Control Study

	Cases	Controls	Total
Exposed	a	b	$a+b$
Unexposed	c	d	$c+d$
Total	$a+c$	$b+d$	$a+b+c+d$

A case-control study begins with a sampling of persons with the disease of interest and individuals without the disease $(a+c$ and $b+d$, respectively). With this approach, the proportion of persons in the study who have the disease is no longer determined by the risk of developing the disease in the source population, but rather by the choice of the investigator. That is, a disease that occurs infrequently in the source population can be over-sampled, so that affected individuals constitute a large proportion of the study sample. This ability to oversample affected individuals is the reason that case-control studies are statistically efficient for the study of rare disease.

For discrete data, the simplest and most common method to determine whether observed differences in proportions between study groups are statistically significant is the chi-square test. The chi-square statistic for a two-by-two table can be expressed as Formula (5.4):

$$\chi^2 = \frac{(ad-bc)^2 n}{(a+b)(c+d)(a+c)(b+d)} \tag{5.4}$$

In a case-control study, the investigator determines the ratio of persons with the disease to persons without it, and thus the proportion of study subjects who have the disease does not provide an estimate of the risk of developing the disease. As shown in the following section, however, an indirect estimate of the incidence rate ratio can still be obtained in a case-control study.

With the notation introduced in Table 5.2, the probability that a case was exposed previously is estimated by Formula(5. 5):

$$\text{Case exposure probability} = \frac{\text{Exposed cases}}{\text{All cases}} = \frac{a}{a+c} \tag{5.5}$$

The odds of exposure for cases represent the probability that a case was exposed divided by the probability that a case was not exposed. The odds then are estimated by Formula (5. 6):

$$\text{Odds of case exposure} = \frac{\text{Exposed cases}}{\text{All cases}} \Big/ \frac{\text{Unexposed cases}}{\text{All cases}} = \frac{a}{a+c} \Big/ \frac{c}{a+c} = \frac{a}{c} \tag{5.6}$$

Similarly, the odds of exposure among controls are estimated by Formula(5. 7):

$$\text{Odds of control exposure} = \frac{b}{b+d} \Big/ \frac{d}{b+d} = \frac{b}{d} \tag{5.7}$$

The odds of exposure for cases divided by the odds of exposure for controls are expressed as the odds ratio (OR). Substituted from the preceding equation, the OR is estimated by Formula (5. 8):

$$\text{Odds ratio} = \frac{\text{Odds of case exposure}}{\text{Odds of control exposure}} = \frac{a}{c} \Big/ \frac{b}{d} = \frac{ad}{bc} \tag{5.8}$$

When incident cases and controls are sampled from the same source population (with selection independent of prior exposure), the OR provides a valid estimate of the incidence rate ratio (see related books). In other words, if properly designed, a case-control study can yield a measure of association between exposure and disease that approximates the incidence rate ratio or relative risk.

5. 3. 2. 2　Construction of the Confidence Intervals

As with the risk ratio, a 95% confidence interval (CI) around the point estimate of the OR can be calculated. The Formula (5. 9) for the confidence interval can be expressed as follows:

$$\ln\text{OR}95\%\text{CI} = \ln\text{OR} \pm 1.96 \sqrt{\text{Var}(\ln\text{OR})} \tag{5.9}$$

This association is unlikely to have occurred by chance alone if the null value of the OR (null value=1) is well outside the 95% confidence interval.

5. 3. 2. 3　Matched Design

In a matched case-control study, the analysis must account for the matched sampling scheme. When one control is matched to each case, summary data can be presented in the format shown in Table 5. 3.

Table 5. 3　Summary Data Format for a Matched Case-Control Study with One Control Per Case

	Cases Exposed	Cases Unexposed	Total
Control Exposed	a	b	$a+b$
Control Unexposed	c	d	$c+d$
Total	$a+c$	$b+d$	$a+b+c+d$

An extension of this basic format can be employed for situations in which the ratio of controls to cases differs from 1 : 1. Although there are four cells in Table 5.3, the entries into this format are quite different from what we find in previous tables. Each entry into Table 5.3 represents not one subject but two (a matched case-control pair). Case-Control pairs that are entered into cells a and d are referred as concordant pairs, because, in these pairs, the exposure status of cases and controls is the same. Case-Control pairs that are entered into cells b and c, in contrast, are referred to as discordant pairs because, in these pairs, the exposure status of cases and controls differs.

In statistics, McNemar's test is a non-parametric method used on nominal data. It is applied to 2×2 contingency tables with a dichotomous trait, with matched pairs of subjects, to determine whether the row and column marginal frequencies are equal ("marginal homogeneity"). The McNemar's test for a 2×2 table can be expressed as Formula (5.10):

$$\chi^2 = \frac{(b-c)^2}{(b+c)} \qquad\qquad (5.10)$$

The OR for a pair-matched case-control study is given by a simple ratio as Formula (5.11):

$$\text{Odds ratio} = \frac{c}{b} \qquad\qquad (5.11)$$

This odds ratio can be interpreted in the same manner as the OR for unmatched studies.

5.3.3 Subgroup and Sensitivity Analysis

A subgroup in the analysis of a study is a technique to control confounding factors that involves the evaluation of the association within homogeneous categories or strata of the confounding variable. It is possible simply to report the unconfounded relative risk estimate for each stratum and calculate a confidence interval around each estimate. It is also useful to calculate a single or summary estimate of the association between exposure and disease, once the effect of the confounding factor (or factors) has been taken into account. A number of statistical methods are available to combine the stratum-specific values into a single overall estimate, all of which calculates a weighted average of effects. The choice of the particular weights depends on the characteristics of data.

The presence or absence of confounding factors should never be assessed by a statistical test of significance. Larger sample size could easily result in a statistically significant association between a confounding factor and the exposure or disease, even though the magnitude may be too small to result in any material amount of a confounding effect. On the other hand, even strong associations that could produce a confounding effect of substantial epidemiologic importance may fail to reach statistical significance with small sample size. Significance testing can be used, however, to evaluate whether the unconfounded estimate of the effect differs from the null value of no association.

Confounding factors are a nuisance effect, resulting in a distortion of the true relationship between the exposure and risk of disease due solely to the particular mix of subjects included in the study. The process of stratification is used to evaluate both confounding factors and effect modification, to control the former, and to describe the latter. The approach to a stratified analysis involves steps as follows:

①Stratify by levels of the potential confounding factor.

②Compute stratum-specific unconfounded relative risk estimates.

③Evaluate the similarity of the stratum-specific estimates by either eyeballing or performing a test of statistical significance.

④If the effect is thought to be uniform, calculate a pooled unconfounded summary estimate using the Mantel-Haenzel odds ratio (OR_{MH}).

⑤Perform hypothesis testing on the unconfounded estimate, using Mantel-Haenszel chi-square and compute the confidence interval.

⑥If the effect is not thought to be uniform (i. e., effect modification is present): Report stratum-specific estimates, results of hypothesis testing, and confidence intervals for each estimate. If desired, calculate a summary unconfounded estimate using a standardized formula.

Another way to deal with the issue of possible assumption violations is to conduct a sensitivity analysis, in which the statistical analysis is systematically repeated, using different assumptions each time, to see how sensitive the statistics changes in the analysis assumptions. In the sensitivity analysis, one may repeat the analysis with different adjustments for uncontrolled confounding, measurement errors, and selection bias, and with different statistical models for computing P-values and confidence limits.

5.3.4　Example

5.3.4.1　Unmatched Design

Example 1

The calculation of the OR can be illustrated by data from a case-control study of lung cancer in which risk associated with smoking was studied. Among 58 lung cancer cases, 22 were smokers, compared with 7 of 93 controls, as summarized in Table 5. 4.

Table 5.4　Summary of Data from the Unmatched Case-Control Study of Lung Cancer and Smoking

	Cases	Controls	Total
Smoking	22	7	29
Non-smoking	36	86	122
Total	58	93	151

The OR for these data is as follows:　Odds ratio$=\dfrac{ad}{bc}=\dfrac{22\times86}{7\times36}=7.5$

In other words, the odds for smokers with lung cancer were over seven times greater than the odds for smokers among controls in this study. To the extent that the OR provides a valid estimate of the incidence rate ratio, it could be calculated from this investigation that smoking increased the likelihood of developing lung cancer more than sevenfold.

5.3.4.2 Matched Design

Example 2

To illustrate the calculation of the OR from a matched study, the results of a hypothetical matched study with 200 matched case-control pairs are shown in Table 5.5.

Table 5.5 Summary of Data from the Matched Case-Control Study of Lung Cancer and Smoking

	Cases Exposed	Cases Unexposed	Total
Controls Exposed	132	5	137
Controls Unexposed	57	6	63
Total	189	11	200

The OR from this study is as follows:

$$\text{Odds ratio} = \frac{c}{b} = \frac{57}{5} = 11.4$$

A 95% confidence interval around the point estimate of the matched OR can be calculated. A formula to calculate an approximate 95% confidence interval is the same as formula in an unmatched case-control study. With the data presented in Table 5.5, the approximately 95% confidence interval for the OR is 4.6 to 28.3. That is, the data from the hypothetical matched case-control study is consistent with a strong to a very strong positive association between the smoking exposure and the development of lung cancer. This association is highly unlikely to have occurred by chance, as the null value of the OR is far outside the 95% confidence interval.

5.4 Types of Bias and the Role of Bias

As with any epidemiologic investigation, the associations derived from a case-control study may not accurately reflect reality due to biases occurring in the course of study design, data collection, or data analysis, etc. Bias is a systematic error in a study that distorts the results and limits the validity of conclusions. Selection bias, information bias and confounding are the three main categories of bias.

5.4.1 Selection Bias

Selection bias can occur whenever the inclusion of cases or controls into the study depends in some way on the exposure of interest. Selection bias is a particular problem in case-control studies since exposure and disease both occurred before subjects are selected for the study. There are a number of situations that can result in this bias. In all of these, the common element is that the relationship between the exposure and disease observed among those who participate in the study is different from that for individuals who would have been eligible to participate but were unwilling or not selected by the investigator. For example, concerns about the existence of selection bias are always raised when response rates are either low or unequal for cases and controls since those who agree to participate are different from those who do not in ways that may be related to the exposure and outcome under investigation. Similarly, if alternate controls are selected to replace those who were originally chosen but could not be contacted or refused to participate, biased estimates could result. There are two particular types of selection bias for a case-control study.

5.4.1.1   Berkson's Bias

It is a type of selection bias which can arise when the sample is taken not from the general population, but from a subpopulation. It was first recognized in case control studies when both cases and controls are sampled from a hospital rather than from the community. When we take the sample, we have to assume that the chance of admission to hospital for the disease is not affected by the presence or absence of the risk factor for that disease. This may not be the case, especially if the risk factor is another disease. This is because people are more likely to be hospitalized if they have two diseases, rather than only one.

5.4.1.2   Neyman's Bias

Also known as prevalence and incidence bias, Neyman's bias is a type of selection bias in a case-control study, which is caused by the prevalent case. If only prevalent cases are used, prognostic factors might be mistakenly inferred as etiological factors.

5.4.2   Information Bias

Information bias, also termed observation bias or measurement bias, results from errors in obtaining information from subjects once they have entered into the study. This type of bias may arise because information on exposure is provided by the participant or a surrogate (proxy) respondent after the onset of disease. Knowledge of the disease status thus may influence the reporting of information by the subject or the recording or interpretation of this information by the investigator. Recall bias and misclassification are two types of information bias that merit particular concern in case-control studies.

Recall bias relates to the difference in the ways that exposure information is remembered or reported by cases, who have experienced an adverse health outcome, and by controls, who have not. When people remember past events, they don't usually have a complete or accurate picture of what happened. In fact, it's been shown that our brains continuously rewrite memories, clouding them with current events, or even editing them completely. Memories can also be distorted by shock at the time of an event, post-traumatic stress disorder or any one of a number of diseases and conditions that affect the brain. Recall bias cannot be corrected after a study has been completed.

Misclassification refers to errors in the categorization of either exposure or disease status. Such errors are inevitable in any study, but the consequences of this type of bias depend on whether the misclassification with respect to one axis (either exposure or disease) is or is not independent of the classification of the other axis. Differential misclassification happens when the information errors differ between groups. In other words, the bias is different for exposed and non-exposed, or between those who have the disease and those do have not. Non-differential classification error happens when the information is incorrect, but is the same across groups. It happens when exposure is unrelated to other variables (including disease), or when the disease is unrelated to other variables (including exposure). Bias introduced by non-differential misclassification is usually predictable (it goes towards the null value), but this is not always the case. Three or more exposure groups (levels) can cause a bias away from the null.

5.4.3　Confounding

Confounding is a distortion (inaccuracy) in the estimated measure of association that occurs when the primary exposure of interest is mixed up with other factors that are associated with the outcome. Methods for addressing potential confounding factors in case-control studies include restriction or matching in the design phase, and stratification and multivariate techniques in the analysis stage. No single method can be considered optimal in every situation. Each has its strengths and limitations that must be carefully considered at the beginning of the study. In most situations, a combination of strategies will provide better insights into the nature of the data and more efficient control of confounding factors than any single approach.

5.5　Advantages and Disadvantages of Case-Control Studies

In this chapter, the basic approach to the design and analysis of case-control studies is presented. A case-control study is a type of observational investigation in which subjects are enrolled on the basis of the presence or absence of a particular disease (e. g. , lung cancer) and are then evaluated to determine their history of prior exposure to risk factors of interest (e. g. , smoking exposure). The advantages and disadvantages of the case-control approach are summarized in Table 5. 6.

Table 5. 6　Advantages and Disadvantages of Case-Control Study

Advantages	Disadvantages
Efficient for the study of rare disease	Risk of the disease cannot be estimated directly
Efficient for the study of chronic disease	Not efficient for the study of rare exposures

(To be continued)

Table 5. 6

Advantages	Disadvantages
Tend to require a smaller sample size than other designs	More susceptible to selection bias than alternative designs
Less expensive than alternative designs	Information on exposure may be less accurate than that available in alternative designs
May be completed more rapidly than alternative designs	

(Jing Chunxia, Zeng Fangfang)

Exercise

Chapter 6   Experimental Studies

As the advanced stage of epidemiological study, experimental studies can produce the highest quality evidence. In observational studies, the investigators simply observe the development of an outcome according to participants' level of exposure. However, in experimental studies, the investigators intervene to change participants' exposure level to determine the effect of the intervention on the outcome. Thus, intervention is the essential difference between observational studies and experimental studies. Experimental studies could be used to evaluate the efficacy and safety of therapeutic or preventive intervention as well as to verify the causal hypothesis.

6.1   Introduction

6.1.1   Definition of Experimental Study

Experimental study, also known as intervention trial, is a branch of epidemiological research in which participants are randomly assigned to experimental and control groups. Then, the intervention of interest is given to participants among the experimental group while a comparison intervention (such as standard intervention or placebo) is given to the controls. The outcomes of participants in different groups is traced and compared to determine the effect of the tested intervention (Figure 6.1).

6.1.2   Features of Experimental Study

6.1.2.1   Prospective Study

In an experimental study, the effect of the intervention is traced after the intervention is given, and thus the experimental study is prospective in nature.

6.1.2.2   Random Allocation

Participants are randomly assigned, or allocated, to the experimental or control groups and neither the investigator nor the participant selects who goes into which group.

6.1.2.3   Comparable Control Group

The control group is similar to the experimental group regarding the distribution of all variables except the intervention. This allows investigators to accurately attribute the difference in the outcome between the experimental and control groups to the different interventions received.

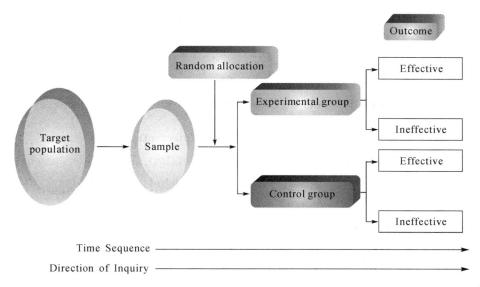

Figure 6. 1   Schematic Diagram of the Basic Principles of Experimental Study

6. 1. 2. 4   Intervention

The characteristic that distinguishes experimental study from observational study is that the participant's level of exposure depends on the purpose of the experimental study. Participants in an experimental study are randomly assigned to the experimental or control group, and they receive the type of intervention according to the group to which they are assigned.

6. 1. 3   Types of Experimental Studies

According to the types of participants and basic units receiving the intervention, experimental studies can be classified into clinical trials, field trials, and community trials.

6. 1. 3. 1   Clinical Trials

In clinical trials, participants are patients with a particular disease and the basic unit receiving intervention is an individual patient. Clinical trials are performed to evaluate the efficacy and safety of therapeutic interventions, such as a drug or surgery, in clinical medicine.

6. 1. 3. 2   Field Trials

In field trials, participants are persons free of disease but likely to develop a certain disease, and the basic unit receiving intervention is an individual person. Field trials are used to evaluate the efficacy and safety of preventive interventions such as vaccines and physical exercise.

6. 1. 3. 3   Community Trials

The community trials are very similar to field trials, except that the basic unit receiving intervention in community trials is a group of people or a community. Community trials are used in situations where it is impossible to perform preventive interventions on the level of an individual. For example, when investigators want to examine the effects of fluoridating water to prevent dental caries, it is impossible to add fluoride to some people's water and not to others'. Thus, whole towns are designated to drink fluoridated water while others are designated to drink non-fluoridated water.

6.1.4　Major Applications of Experimental Study

6.1.4.1　To Evaluate the Efficacy and Safety of Intervention

The main application of experimental study is to evaluate the effect (including efficacy and safety) of the intervention of interest (including therapeutic and preventive intervention).

6.1.4.2　To Verify the Causal Hypothesis

In experimental studies, investigators intervene to change participants' levels of exposure. Ethical considerations demand that participants not be exposed to risk factors. Therefore, when experimental studies are used to verify a causal hypothesis, the possible risk factor should be eliminated from participants in the experimental group.

6.2　Clinical Trial

6.2.1　Definition of Clinical Trial

As mentioned earlier, the clinical trial is one type of experimental study used to determine the efficacy and safety of therapeutic intervention among patients with a particular disease. In the clinical trial, patients with a particular disease are randomly allocated into experimental and control groups. Patients in the experimental group receive the tested therapeutic intervention, and patients in the control group receive a standard treatment or placebo. Efficacy and safety information is collected prospectively. A comparison is then made between the experimental group and the control group. Results from clinical trials could provide solid support for clinical treatment decisions, and the evidence generated from clinical trials has promoted the development and progress of evidence-based medicine.

Most clinical trials are applied to evaluate the efficacy and safety of a new drug, and strict procedures are used to assess new drugs. In addition to pre-clinical pharmacological and toxicological evaluations, the efficacy and safety of a new drug should be rigorously assessed using different phases of clinical trials, which may be categorized into four phases.

6.2.1.1　Phase Ⅰ trials

These trials are usually performed in a small number of volunteers to determine the pharmacokinetics and side effects of a new drug. Phase I trials provide a reference for determining dosage regimens. Volunteers could be healthy persons or patients with the target disease.

6.2.1.2　Phase Ⅱ trials

These trials are usually carried out in several hundred patients (usually $100-300$) with the target disease to preliminarily assess the efficacy and safety of a tested drug. Phase Ⅱ trials provide evidence for the study design and dosage regimen of phase Ⅲ trials. In phase Ⅱ trials, multiple forms of clinical trial design, including blind randomized controlled trials (RCTs), could be applied to achieve the goal.

6.2.1.3　Phase Ⅲ trials

These large-scale RCTs (usually including $1000-3000$ patients) are conducted to further verify the efficacy and safety of a tested drug, and most of the clinical trials belong to this phase. Since the sample size required is relatively large, patients are usually recruited from multiple centers. If the tested drug passes phase Ⅲ trials, it can be approved and licenzed for marketing.

6.2.1.4　Phase IV trials

Also known as post-marketing surveillance, these trials are essentially not RCTs. Phase IV trials are performed to determine the efficacy and safety of a new drug under widely used conditions, for the following reasons: patients in clinical trials are selected strictly according to inclusion and exclusion criteria, so the efficacy and safety of the drug among patients not included in the trial is unclear; clinical trials are usually conducted over a relatively short period, and thus the long-term efficacy and safety must be monitored; uncommon side effects cannot be observed in clinical trials with relatively small sample sizes; the results of clinical trials must be further verified in real-world settings. Taken together, phase IV trials could provide valuable evidence on the risk and benefit among general or special populations and help optimize the dosage regimen of a new drug.

6.2.2　Basic Principles of Clinical Trials

Clinical trials could be categorized into randomized and non-randomized controlled trials according to whether the patients are randomly allocated. The majority of clinical trials are RCTs, which should comply with the following principles.

6.2.2.1　Randomization

Patients are allocated into groups by chance. The use of randomization could yield similar groups at the start of an investigation, for both known and unknown variables.

6.2.2.2　Control

In a clinical trial, the control group is set to differentiate the specific effect from the non-specific effect of the tested therapeutic intervention.

6.2.2.3　Blinding

Blinding is a measure used to keep groups of people (patients, evaluators, and analysts) involved in a clinical trial unaware of patients' treatment assignment, with the aim of minimizing bias resulting from the possible effect of psychological factors.

6.2.2.4　Replication

Replication is another measure used to eliminate the non-specific effect of the intervention. Since the conclusion of a clinical trial is based on statistical analysis and two types of error might occur, clinical trials should be carried out with adequate sample sizes to verify the effect of the therapeutic intervention tested.

6.2.3　Design and Implementation of Clinical Trial

Since RCTs have been widely accepted as the "gold standard" for evaluating the efficacy and safety of an intervention, this section introduces the design and implementation of RCTs.

6.2.3.1　Determining the Purpose of the Clinical Trial

Clinical trials are mainly used to assess the efficacy and safety of therapeutic interventions such as drugs and surgery. The purpose of a clinical trial is usually to determine the absolute value and relative value of therapeutic interventions of interest. The main components of a clinical trial include patients, the intervention, comparator, and outcome, which are commonly expressed as PICO. The design of a clinical trial is mainly concerned with the specification of these four points. For example, a clinical trial might be performed to examine whether vitamin D supplementation could be used to treat symptomatic knee osteoarthritis in patients with low 25-hydroxyvitamin D levels compared to a placebo. The patients in this study should be patients with symptomatic knee osteoarthritis and low levels of 25-hydroxyvitamin D, and the intervention to be tested is vitamin D supplementation; the comparator is the placebo, and the outcome should be some variables used to measure the efficacy and safety of vitamin D supplementation.

6.2.3.2　Selecting Patients

In a clinical trial, participants are patients with a particular disease. Patient inclusion and exclusion criteria should be specified in advance, based on the comprehensive consideration of scientificity, feasibility, and ethical issues. These criteria determine who will or will not be included in the clinical trial. When selecting patients, we should include patients who are more likely to respond well to treatment. We should consider whether we have to restrict the severity and stage of the disease, previous treatment history, contaminant drug use, and other similar factors. Since the patients must be followed to assess efficacy and safety, we should include patients who could adhere to the treatment and be traced effectively. In addition, groups of people who are particularly vulnerable should be excluded, such as children, elderly people, and pregnant and breastfeeding women. After screening patients according to the inclusion and exclusion criteria, eligible patients should be randomly allocated into the intervention group and the control group. In a clinical trial, the most commonly used randomization methods include simple randomization, block randomization, and stratified randomization. The main goal of randomization is to minimize confounding bias by achieving comparable treatment groups in terms of the even distribution of known and unknown confounding factors. When the confounding bias is minimized, differences in outcome between treatment groups at the end of the study are more likely due to differences in treatments received. In general, the probability of achieving balance in the number of participants for each treatment groups is in proportion to the sample size.

Simple randomization is the most straightforward way to allocate patients into different treatment groups and can be accomplished by tossing a coin, drawing lots, or using a random number table. When the sample size is small and many factors are associated with the outcome of the therapeutic intervention, block randomization can be applied. In block randomization, patients are divided into blocks, in which with the same number of patients have similar characteristics such as age, sex, disease severity, and ethnicity, etc. Patients in the same block are then randomly allocated into different groups using the simple randomization approach. In stratified randomization, patients are categorized into several homogenous strata according to one factor (such as age, sex, or body mass index) associated with the effect of the therapeutic intervention. Patients in the same strata are then assigned into different groups using the simple randomization method.

6.2.3.3 Sample Size Estimation

Since sampling error is inversely proportional to sample size, the aim of sample size estimation is to obtain a relatively small sample to reach a relatively solid conclusion. The sample size of a clinical trial is determined by the following factors: the expected magnitude of difference in outcome between groups; the required type I error level, usually expressed as the level of α; the required type II error level, usually expressed as the level of β. The value of $(1-\beta)$ refers to the study's ability to detect a significant difference at the level of α, using a one-tailed or two-tailed test. According to the types of outcome variables, different formulas are applied to calculate the corresponding sample size.

①When the outcome variable is qualitative, it is usually expressed as rate, such as effective rate, death rate, and case-fatality rate. The formula (6.1) is as follows:

$$N=\frac{(Z_{\alpha/2}\sqrt{2\,\overline{p}\,\overline{q}}+Z_{\beta}\,\sqrt{p_0 q_0+p_1 q_1}\,)^2}{(p_1-p_0)^2} \tag{6.1}$$

N—the calculated sample size; $Z_{\alpha/2}$—the constant from the standard normal distribution depending on the value of α; Z_{β}—the constant from the standard normal distribution depending on the value of β; p_1—the expected event rate in the experimental group; p_0—the expected event rate in the control group; q_1-1-p_1; q_0-1-p_0; $\overline{p}-(p_0+p_1)/2$; $\overline{q}=1-\overline{p}$.

②When the outcome variable is quantitative, such as height and weight, the calculation Formula (6.2) is as follows:

$$N=\frac{2(Z_{\alpha/2}+Z_{\beta})^2\sigma^2}{d^2} \tag{6.2}$$

N—the calculated sample size; $Z_{\alpha/2}$—the constant from the standard normal distribution depending on the value of α; Z_β—the constant from the standard normal distribution depending on the value of β; σ—the estimated standard deviation; d—the difference in means between groups.

It should be noted that the N is the estimated number of patients for one group. If two groups with the same number of patients are required, the total sample size should be double N. In addition, since the clinical trial is essentially a prospective study, loss to follow-up is inevitable. Thus, we should include more patients than the estimated number, and we usually add approximately 10—15 percent more.

6. 2. 3. 4 Setting Control

The rationale for establishing a control group is to differentiate the specific effect from the non-specific effect of the tested intervention. The non-specific effect includes unpredictable outcomes, regression toward the mean, the effect of other factors associated with the outcome, the Hawthorne effect, and the placebo effect. The Hawthorne results from a subject altering behavior because he or she is being observed, regardless of experimental manipulation. For example, one study of hand-washing among medical staff found that when the study subjects knew they were being watched, compliance with hand-washing was 55 percent greater than when they perceived they were not being watched. The placebo effect is the positive effect on a person's health owing to the person's belief in the benefit of medical treatment and their expectation of feeling better. The commonly used control types in a clinical trial include standard control, placebo control, crossover control, mutual control, and self-control.

(1)Standard Control

Also known as positive control, the standard (i. e. , the most commonly used or the most effective) treatment is given to patients in the control group, in accordance with the ethical requirement of clinical studies. Thus, this is also the most commonly used control type.

(2)Placebo Control

Also known as negative control, the placebo is given to patients in the control group. A placebo is a substance or treatment of no therapeutic value; it must resemble the tested treatment in terms of appearance, shape, taste, smell, and mode of delivery. Commonly used placebos include inert tablets (like sugar pills), inert injections (like saline), sham surgery, and other procedures. Since placebos contain no active pharmaceutical component, their use is ethically problematic. The placebo can be applied only when no curative measure is available or the use of placebo has no effect on the prognosis of disease.

(3)Crossover Control

This is a specific type of control derived from the crossover trial study design. In the two-period crossover trial, patients receive both treatments (tested therapeutic intervention and control therapeutic intervention) in successive order. For each patient, the order in which treatments are received—tested therapeutic intervention followed by control therapeutic intervention, or vice versa—is determined randomly. A washout period is required between the two periods, with the goal of minimizing carryover effects, including pharmacological and psychological effects, of the treatment received in the first period to the treatment received in the second period. In this type of trial, comparisons can be made within the same patient, and the effect of the order of treatment can be evaluated. However, this type of trial requires more time, and the loss to follow-up rate might be high. The crossover trial design is typically used when the condition being investigated is chronic and treatment is being evaluated for short-term relief of symptoms rather than provide a cure.

(4)Mutual Control

When multiple therapeutic interventions are simultaneously tested in one trial, no specific control group is required. The multiple arms (groups of patients receiving different therapeutic interventions) can be mutually compared when the data is analyzed.

(5)Self-Control

Tested and control therapeutic intervention can be compared within the same patient, and each participant can act as his or her own control. This includes the comparison of before and after the tested therapeutic intervention was received, as well as the comparison of tested and control therapeutic intervention given on the left and right hand, foot, eye, or limb of the same person.

6.2.3.5　Data Collection

In clinical trials, a case report form (CRF) should be designed to collect related data according to the trial's goals. Data, including baseline and follow-up data, should be carefully recorded in the CRF, and the same procedure should be adopted for each patient in the entire process to ensure that the data collected for each study group is consistent.

Baseline data, namely the data collected when the patient enters a clinical trial, often comprises demographic characteristics, clinical characteristics, drug use data (previous and present drug use), behavior and lifestyle data, personal and family history of disorders, physical and laboratory test data, and imaging data. Baseline data is collected to know the basic characteristics of patients included in the study, providing virtual information about the generalizability of the clinical trial. Furthermore, baseline data between the intervention group and control group can be compared to verify whether randomization has achieved reasonable comparability between the two groups in terms of confounding factors associated with the concerned outcomes of the clinical trial.

During follow-up, the following data should be collected: treatment compliance, change in confounding factors, and outcomes. Treatment compliance refers to the extent to which the patient has complied with the allocated treatment, so detailed information about the treatment (dose, frequency, route of administration, and time of administration, etc.) should be recorded carefully. It is common for a patient to change or discontinue his or her assigned treatment for objective or subjective reasons. Since some confounding factors might be time-varying covariates, attention should also be paid to changes in the confounding factors. Outcomes are any effect of the tested intervention. These effects could be categorized into two aspects, efficacy and safety, and both are indispensable. Several points should be noted when outcomes are determined. First, based on the consideration from the various people (patients, clinicians, health care providers, etc.) involved in a clinical trial, multiple outcomes should be selected to comprehensively assess the effect of the tested intervention. For example, the investigators might be more concerned about improvement in the clinical symptoms and laboratory test results, while patients might pay much more attention to physical function. In general, a few (in most cases only one) primary and multiple secondary outcomes are determined. Second, quantitative and objective variables are preferable to qualitative and subjective ones. Finally, measurement of the outcomes should be defined in advance and should be kept consistent throughout the entire process.

6.2.3.6　The Application of Blinding

Blinding, sometimes known as masking, is a measure used to ensure that persons (patients, evaluators, and analysts) involved in clinical trial are unaware of the treatment assigned to patients, with the goal of minimizing bias resulting from psychological factors. Placebos with the same characteristics (including appearance, shape, taste, smell, and mode of delivery) of the tested treatment are commonly used as an inert treatment to achieve blinding. In a single-blind trial, only the patients are unaware of their assigned treatment, which is particularly important when the outcome is measured subjectively, such as in trials investigating pain relief. For example, if the patient knows that he or she is receiving a new drug and is suspicious of this new drug, the patient might be more likely to report worse outcomes and or withdraw from the trial in advance. Since the evaluators' knowledge of the treatment assigned would also significantly distort the results, the double-blind is the most commonly used clinical trial, in which both patients and evaluators are unaware of the patients' assigned treatment. For example, if the evaluators are aware of patients' assigned treatment, they might show different attitudes toward patients in different treatment groups. A triple-blind trial is one in which the patients' treatment assignment is unknown to patients, evaluators, and data analysts.

However, blinding is not always feasible or necessary. For interventions with typical side effects and some special types of intervention such as behavior change or surgery, it might be impossible or unethical to mask the treatment assignment of patients. This scenario is considered an open-label trial. Furthermore, the need for blinding is also determined by whether the outcome is subjectively measured. If the outcome may be objectively measured, such as results based on a urine or blood sample test, the use of blinding is not necessary.

6.2.3.7　Data Analysis

The integrity and validity of data should be checked before data analysis. Statistical analysis includes statistical description and statistical inference. Statistical indexes, tables, and charts could be applied when performing statistical description. The baseline characteristics of eligible and randomized patients should be described in detail, and the use of a flow diagram of the progress through the trial phases (including recruitment, treatment alloca- tion, follow-up, and data analysis) is strongly recommended. Statistical inference is per- formed to estimate the population parameter (effective rate in most cases) based on sample statistics and to deduce whether there is a significant difference in baseline characteristics and outcome measures (such as the effective rate and the adverse event rate) between differ- ent treatment groups.

The most commonly used indicators for clinical trials include the effective rate, the cure rate, the case fatality rate, the adverse event rate, the survival rate, the relative risk reduc- tion (RRR), the absolute risk reduction (ARR), and the number needed to treat (NNT). NNT, an indicator developed to help practitioners understand the results of clinical trials relevant to their practice, is the reciprocal of the ARR in the outcome measurements be- tween the experimental and control groups. For example, if the rate of adverse outcome in the control group is 8 percent and 3 percent in experimental group, the NNT $= 1 / (8\% - 3\%) = 20$. This means that the treatment of 20 patients with the tested therapeutic interven- tion will result in one less adverse outcome than if they received the control intervention.

In addition, it should be noted that some patients might be lost to follow-up or don't comply with assigned treatment during the trial, and thus intention-to-treat (ITT) analysis or per-protocol (PP) analysis methods could be applied. In the ITT analysis method, all pa- tients are analyzed and outcome measurements are compared between different treatment groups based on the group to which patients are originally randomly allocated, regardless of whether they complete the trial or comply with the assigned treatment. ITT analysis usually leads to underestimating the true effect of tested therapeutic intervention compared with the control, because it includes patients who are non-adherent to or deviated from the protocol. PP analysis, sometimes known as "on treatment" analysis, uses only data from patients who adhere to the assigned treatment. Thus, patients who do not comply with the assigned treatment are excluded from PP analysis, and this usually results in overestimating the true effect of the tested therapeutic intervention compared with the control. Of note, a confound- ing bias might occur when PP analysis is conducted. Since patients who do not comply with their allocated treatment protocol are excluded, the original comparability of the treatment groups in baseline characteristics achieved after randomization may not be maintained. In conclusion, ITT and PP analysis should be done simultaneously to reach a solid conclusion based on the comparison of results derived from these two different strategies.

6.2.4   Bias of Clinical Trials

RCTs have been widely accepted as the gold standard for evaluating the efficacy and safety of therapeutic intervention because several measures are incorporated to minimize bi- as. Randomization is mainly used to minimize confounding bias by obtaining treatment groups with similar baseline characteristics. Blinding is mainly employed to overcome information bias caused by patients' knowledge about the treatment assignments from different groups involved in the clinical trial. In addition, RCTs are essentially prospective studies, so the cause precedes the effect, which is in accordance with the temporal sequence from cause to effect. However, it should be noted that RCTs are also vulnerable to some types of bias.

6.2.4.1   Loss to Follow-up Bias

As a prospective study, patients in RCTs must be followed to determine the efficacy and safety of the tested therapeutic intervention, making the loss to follow-up inevitable. During the trial, patients might be lost to follow-up due to several reasons, such as: moving away; dying from other diseases or accidents; being lost to contact; losing interest in the trial; being busy or ill, etc. If there is a systematic difference in characteristics associated with the outcome between patients who are lost to follow-up and those who complete the study, bias might occur. Several measures should be employed to control loss to follow-up bias: when selecting patients, those who are more likely to be followed well should receive top consideration; patients should be briefed on all the aspects (including the aims, methods, and possible benefit and risk, etc.) of the trial to obtain their cooperation; blinding should be applied since bias might result from their knowledge of treatment assignment.

6.2.4.2   Co-intervention and Contamination Bias

Co-intervention bias can occur if patients in the experimental group receive other effective treatment, and this will lead to overestimating the effect of the tested therapeutic intervention. When patients in the control group receive the experimental intervention, the resultant contamination bias can result in underestimating the effect of the tested therapeutic intervention. These two types of bias stem from patients not following protocol for their assigned treatment. The following measures should be applied to control such bias: blinding should be applied because seeking or providing other treatments might be due to patients' or care providers' knowledge of assigned treatment; patients should be treated strictly according to the protocol.

6.3   Advantages and Disadvantages of Experimental Study

6.3.1   Advantages

①The use of randomization ensures the comparability of participants in the experimental and control groups, which could minimize the influence of confounding bias.

②The experimental study is essentially a prospective study, multiple approaches including randomization and blinding are applied to control bias, and thus experimental study design could produce the epidemiological evidence with the highest quality compared with other epidemiological study designs.

③The experimental study could be employed to investigate the natural history of a disease and to evaluate the associations between one intervention and multiple outcomes.

6.3.2 Disadvantages

①The successful design and performance of experimental study is relatively difficult, which is seldom achieved in daily practice.

②Since an estimated number of participants are required and the participants must be followed up to determine the efficacy and safety of the tested intervention, the cost of an experimental study in terms of human labor, time, and money is a relatively high.

③The generalizability of experimental study might be limited due to the selection of participants according to inclusion and exclusion criteria.

④Similar to a cohort study, loss to follow-up is inevitable in an experimental study, so results should be interpreted with caution.

⑤An ethical issue might arise if the control group is given inappropriate intervention such as a placebo. Standard control should be used preferentially, and the placebo should only be adopted when no curative measure is available or the use of placebo has no effect on the prognosis of the disease.

6.4 Ethical Issues of Experimental Study

Since experimental study is one type of medical research in which human subjects are taken as participants and human intervention is given, much more attention should be paid to ethical issues. The ethical requirements for medical research involving human subjects throughout the world are defined by the Declaration of Helsinki (DoH), issued by the World Medical Association (WMA). The first version of the DoH was adopted in 1964, and subsequently the DoH has been amended seven times, most recently at the General Assembly in October 2013. Experimental study should be carried out in accordance with the DoH, and several points should be emphasized. The design and implementation of the experimental study must be clearly depicted and justified in a research protocol that includes a statement of ethical considerations and how the principles in the DoH are addressed. The research protocol must be approved by the appropriate ethics committee before the study begins. When selecting the type of control, standard control (the most effective or the most commonly used intervention) is preferred to protect the health rights of participants. The placebo control should only be used when no curative measure is available or the use of a placebo has no effect on the prognosis of the disease. Every precaution must be taken to protect the privacy of research subjects and the confidentiality of their personal information. In addition, informed consent must be obtained from every participant. This implies that all participants must be informed of the aims, methods, the anticipated benefits and potential risks of the study, the discomfort it may entail, post-study provisions, and any other relevant aspects of the study. With this information, potential participants can make an informed decision as to whether or not they wish to take part in the study.

(Cen Han, Zhang Lina, Jenny Bowman, Zhao Jinshun)

Exercise

Chapter 7   Causal Inference

Causal inference is the quantification of the effect of an exposure or treatment on an outcome. This includes the thought processes and methods that assess whether a cause-effect relation exists, or that estimate the size of a causal relationship using some measure of effect. In epidemiology, causal inference is often conducted under the potential outcome or counterfactual models.

7.1   Concept of Cause

A cause brings about an effect or a result. In medicine, an understanding of the causes of disease is important for health, not only for prevention but also for diagnosis and applying correct treatments. The first understanding of the causes of disease came from studying infectious diseases in the population. Fracastoro proposed that a specific disease was associated with a living contagion in the 16th century. Koch proposed that a disease has a specific causative agent (single etiology).

In 1882, the microscope was invented, enabling scientists to find pathogens. That same year, Robert Koch(with contributions of F. G. Jacob Henle) promulgated a set of criteria for determining whether an infectious agent is the cause of disease. Koch devised his postulates with the assumption that a particular disease has one cause and a particular cause results in one disease. He stated that four postulates should be met before a causative relationship can be accepted:

①The bacteria must be present in every case of the disease.

②The bacteria must be isolated from the host with the disease and grown in pure culture.

③The specific disease must be reproduced when a pure culture of the bacteria is inoculated into a healthy susceptible host.

④The bacteria must be recoverable from the experimentally infected host.

Koch's postulates had a great impact on the development of etiological theory, especially during the early years of epidemiology when interest was focused on acute infectious diseases. The theory considered the pathogen, but failed to consider the body and environmental conditions. For most chronic or non-infectious diseases, a single cause cannot be simply established by postulates, and often many factors appear to act together to cause disease.

Later, the theory of multifactorial causation was proposed stating disease is associated with many factors (multifactorial causation), such as hosts, environments, behaviors, and psychological and social factors. Probability was applied to this theory.

Lilienfeld defined the cause of a disease as something that may increase the chance of developing a disease. When one or a few factors do not exist, disease frequency will drop. This definition was based on probability.

K. J. Rothman, in his textbook *Modern Epidemiology*, defined the cause of a specific disease as an antecedent event, condition, or characteristic necessary for the occurrence of the disease at the moment it occurred, given that other conditions are fixed. In other words, the cause of a disease is an event, condition, or characteristic that precedes the disease onset, and, had the event, condition, or characteristic been different in a specified way, the disease either would not have occurred at all or would not have occurred until some later time. This understanding is a simplistic misbelief if it emphasizes "one cause—one effect". Most outcomes are caused by a chain or web consisting of many component causes. But Rothman explained that the sufficient cause of a disease could not contribute to a single factor and introduced the concept of component causes. What is a sufficient cause? What is a model of sufficient cause? These concepts will be explained in the following sections.

In epidemiology, the term "risk factor" is preferred to the term "cause". A risk factor is an attribute or exposure associated with an increased risk of disease or other specified outcomes. Risk factors could be genetic factors, environmental exposures, aspects of personal lifestyles, and/or social characteristics. A risk factor may be a cause of disease, but it also may be a non-causal characteristic associated with a disease.

"Causality" refers to the process relating causes to the effects they produce, and much of an epidemiologist's work attempts to establish causality. Epidemiological studies can provide powerful evidence on causality, but epidemiological evidence alone is rarely sufficient to establish causality.

7. 2 Cause Models

The cause theory has changed accordingly with the in-depth study of the concept of cause. The relationship between cause and disease can be expressed through the cause model, which is a concise relational graph that provides causal frames and paths.

7. 2. 1 Classical Models

7. 2. 1. 1 Triangle Model

The triangle model, also called the triangle of epidemiology, holds that the occurrence of a disease is the result of the combined action of the host, environment, and pathogens (Figure 7. 1). Under normal circumstances, people present a healthy state through the interaction of these three elements to maintain a dynamic balance. Once one element changes and exceeds what the triangle balance can maintain, the balance is destroyed and people will suffer from disease. This model considers the three factors of morbidity, but it is difficult to explain chronic and non-communicable diseases due to the absence of specific etiology.

7.2.1.2 Wheel Model

The wheel model emphasizes the close relationship between host and environment. The host occupies the position of the wheel axis, in which the genetic material plays an important role. The peripheral wheel represents the environment, which includes the biological, physical, chemical, and social environment (see Figure 7.2). The organism lives in the environment, while the disease exists in the organism and the environment. The parts of the wheel model structure are flexible and vary in size with different diseases.

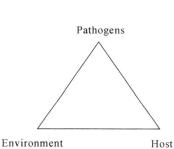

Figure 7.1   Triangle of Epidemiology

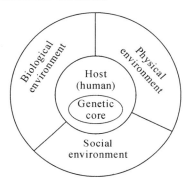

Figure 7.2   Wheel Model in Epidemiology

7.2.1.3 Webs of Causation Model

Multi-etiology theory holds that diseases occur as a result of the combined action of various factors, which can act independently or synergize or antagonize each other. Factors can cause and affect each other, leading to the diversity of disease occurrence. Different pathogenic factors and diseases are connected in different ways; that is, multiple chains of causation are interlinked to form a web of causation. The web of causation model can provide a complete path of causation. The advantages of this model are it's clear and specific expression, it is highly systematic, and it provides a good description of complex causality.

7.2.2   Necessary Cause and Sufficient Cause

Several types of causes can be distinguished. According to Last's Dictionary of Epidemiology (Last, 2001), a cause is termed "necessary" when it must always precede an effect, although the effect needs not to be the sole result of the cause. A cause is termed "sufficient" when it inevitably initiates or produces an effect.

In reality, any given cause may be necessary, sufficient, neither, or both. Many factors that contribute to disease occurrence are neither necessary nor sufficient. For example, tobacco smoking is a cause of lung cancer, but by itself, it is not a sufficient cause, as demonstrated by the fact that smoking will not cause lung cancer in every one. On the other hand, the development of lung cancer could not be fully explained by smoking.

Hence, as has long been recognized in epidemiology, a need exists to develop a more refined conceptual model to serve as a starting point in discussions of causation. In particular, such a model should address problems of multifactorial causation, confounding, the interdependence of effects, direct and indirect effects, levels of causation, and systems or webs of causation (MacMahon and Pugh, 1967; Susser, 1973). We will describe the sufficient-cause model (or sufficient-component cause model), which has been proven useful in elucidating certain concepts in individual mechanisms of causation.

7.2.3 Sufficient-Cause Model

For many people, early causal thinking persists in attempts to find a single cause to explain observed phenomena. But experience and reasoning show that the cause of any effect must consist of a constellation of components that act in concert (Mill, 1862; Mackie, 1965). A characteristic of the naive concept of causation is the assumption of a one-to-one correspondence between the observed cause and effect.

7.2.3.1 A Sufficient Cause on the Basis of the Sufficient-Cause Model

Under the definition of cause proposed by K. J. Rothman, if someone is suffering from clinical tuberculosis (TB), there may be many causes. These causes might include the characteristics of *Mycobacterium tuberculosis* strains, the number of infecting bacilli, an environment of dry air, the existence of small droplet nuclei containing *Mycobacterium tuberculosis*, and a number of patient characteristics including genetic susceptibility, immune status, living conditions and socioeconomic status, access to preventive treatment for latent infection, and so forth. The constellation of causes required for this patient to develop clinical tuberculosis at this time can be depicted with the sufficient cause diagrammed in Figure 7.3. Sufficient cause refers to a complete causal mechanism, a minimal set of conditions and events that are sufficient for the outcome to occur; "minimal" here implies that all the conditions or events are necessary. The circle in the figure comprises four segments, which respectively represent a causal component that must be present or has occurred for the person to develop TB. The first component, labeled A, represents *Mycobacterium tuberculosis*. The second component, labeled B, represents small droplet nuclei. The third component, labeled C, represents immune status. The fourth component, labeled U, represents the set of unknown factors. For etiologic effects such as the causation of disease, many and possibly all the components of a sufficient cause may be unknown (Rothman, 1976a).

In disease etiology, a sufficient cause is a set of conditions sufficient to ensure an outcome will occur. All the component causes in the sufficient cause must be present. None is superfluous, which means that blocking the contribution of any component cause prevents the sufficient cause from acting.

7.2.3.2 A Necessary Cause on the Basis of the Sufficient-Cause Model

Consider again the role of small droplet nuclei in causing TB. Small droplet nuclei may play a causal role in this sufficient cause but not in others. A small number of instances have occurred where TB was acquired through contact with broken skin. That to say the small droplet nuclei is a component cause of clinical TB does not, however, imply that every person contacting the droplet nuclei will develop TB. Nor does it imply that the person who does not contact the droplet nuclei will not develop TB. There may be other sufficient causes by which a person could suffer clinical TB. Under this view, each of factors noted above can be a component of a sufficient causal model, and there may be several sufficient causal models of clinical tuberculosis. Each such sufficient cause would be depicted by its own diagram like Figure 7.3.

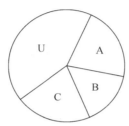

Figure 7.3 Depiction of the constellation of component causes that constitute a sufficient cause for a patient of TB at a particular time (built on Rothman's figure, 2008). The diagram contains four components: A, B, C, and U representing *Mycobacterium tuberculosis*, small droplet nuclei, immune status, and the set of unknown factors, respectively.

One circle, or pie, depicts a sufficient causal model, which represents the certain causal mechanism in Figure 7.4. Here the letters A, B, C, and so on respectively represent different factors. Figure 7.4a shows a certain disease has sufficient causes containing components A, B and C (U is an unknown factor); that is, when A, B, and C exist in a certain person, the disease will inevitably occur (of course, the unknown factor must also be considered). In the same way, Figure 7.4b and c show the other sufficient causes. Each cause is "necessary" and "sufficient" to produce the effect, particularly when the cause is an observable action or event that takes place near in time to the effect. If any of the component causes appears in every sufficient cause, then that component cause is called a necessary component cause. The term *necessary cause* is therefore reserved for a component cause under the sufficient-cause model. Factor A appears in all three sufficient-cause models in Figure 7.4; therefore, factor A is a necessary cause. Rothman explained the example of hip fracture in his textbook and showed that one could label a component cause with the requirement that one must have a hip to suffer a hip fracture. Every sufficient cause that leads to hip fracture must have that component cause present because to fracture a hip, one must have a hip to fracture.

In a word, any factor that appears in at least one sufficient-cause model is called a component cause, and any component cause that appears in all sufficient models is a necessary cause. Each sufficient cause has an independent effect on the occurrence of the disease in a population. Rothman's sufficient-cause model helps us to understand the multifactorial nature of disease etiology and the biological interrelations among these causes.

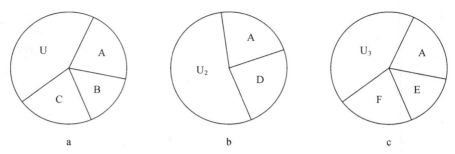

Figure 7.4　Depictions of Three Sufficient-Cause Models of Certain Diseases

7.2.3.3　The Complementary Component Causes

The concept of complementary component causes is useful in epidemiology applications. For each component cause in a sufficient cause, the set of other component causes in that sufficient cause are the complementary component causes. For example, in Figure 7.3, the component cause is A (*Mycobacterium tuberculosis*) with complementary component causes B, C, and U. For the component cause C (immune status), the complementary component causes are A, B, and U.

7.3　Causal Inference in Epidemiology

Figure 7.5 shows the epidemiological process of ascertaining the cause of a disease. The first step,"descriptive study", and the third step,"test hypothesis", are discussed in other chapters. Mill's canons in generating hypotheses and Hill's criteria in causal inference are discussed here.

Epidemiological causal inference includes three steps: ①propose cause clues and establish hypotheses by descriptive studies, such as cross-sectional studies and ecological studies; ②test hypotheses with analytical epidemiological studies, such as case-control studies and cohort studies, and experimental studies; ③infer whether the association between disease and exposure is causal.

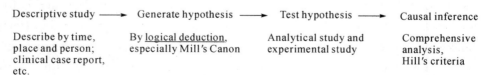

Figure 7.5　The Epidemiological Process of Ascertaining the Cause of Disease

7.3.1　Hypothetico-Deductive Method

In forming an etiological hypothesis, the hypothetico-deductive method and Mill's canon are two commonly used inference methods.

The hypothetico-deductive method, proposed by the Dutch physicist Christiaan Huygens (1629—1695), gave a strong impetus to the development of modern science. Deduction here refers to the empirical facts to be observed, which can be deduced from the hypothesis relative to the background knowledge. The specific individual facts are derived from the general hypothesis via deductive inference. An inductive inference is also required to deduce that, because a fact is true, a general assumption is also true.

①Since Hypothesis (H) is assumed, evidence (E) is deduced (deductive inference).

②Since E is obtained, H is supported in reverse (inductive inference).

In the study of the causal relationship between HBV and primary liver cancer, it is assumed that persistent HBV infection leads to primary liver cancer (H). Based on this hypothesis and relevant background knowledge, the following empirical evidence can be deduced: HBV infection rate in the liver cancer group is higher than that in the control group (E1); an HBV infected cohort has a higher incidence of liver cancer than the control group (E2); after controlling HBV infection, the incidence of liver cancer decreases (E3). If the evidence E1, E2, and E3 are true, the hypothesis H is also supported inductively with corresponding strengths.

7.3.2 Mill's Canons

Mill's canon represents logical strategies developed by John Stuart Mill, an English philosopher, for generating hypotheses between the factor (e. g. , a circumstance) and the phenomenon (e. g. , an outcome or effect). Other scientists also improved the canons. These strategies described are especially pertinent to epidemiology.

7.3.2.1 The Method of Agreement

If two or more instances of an outcome under investigation have one factor in common, the factor, in which alone all the instances agree, may be the cause of the given outcome. The method consists of a search for a single factor common to several situations in which the same event occurred. It detects a cause as a necessary condition. For example, leptospirosis epidemic is the outcome (A=leptospirosis case) and contacting infected water is the common factor (a=water contact), as shown in Figure 7.6. We can generate a hypothesis that infected water may be the cause of the leptospirosis.

Event(D)	Exposure
Subjects 1	ABC — — — — — — abc
Subjects 2	ADE — — — — — — aed
Subjects 3	AFG — — — — — — afg

Figure 7.6 Schematic Diagram of the Method of Agreement

7.3.2.2 The Method of Difference

A second test to determine whether a given factor plays a causal role requires us to take away that factor, holding everything else constant, and to see whether the effect still oc-curs. Mill called this the method of difference. In testing the efficacy of new medicine, for example, two carefully matched groups would be used. One group would get the drug, and the other would get a placebo. The only difference between the groups would be the pres-ence or absence of the drug so that any difference in the results could be attributed to that factor. In summary, if all controls are alike except that the consequence being studied is on-ly present when a certain condition is also present, then that condition may be the cause.

7.3.2.3　The Method of Concomitant Variation

A phenomenon varying in any manner whenever another phenomenon varies in some manner, is either a cause or an effect of that phenomenon, or relates to it through some fact of causation. In other words, this interaction indicates a dose-response relationship.

7.3.2.4　The Method of Residuals

If several effects with several different causes all occur together and some of the causes are already known to cause some of the effects, the residue of the effect is brought about by the residual of the cause. For example, a certain dermatitis occurred in Shanghai in 1972. In the end, the larva of *Euproctis similis* was identified as the cause after ruling out water, food, air pollutants, and other possible causes. As a result, dermatitis was defined in 1972 as euproctis similis dermatitis.

7.3.2.5　The Method of Analogy

An analogy is a comparison of two things to explain something unfamiliar through its similarities to something familiar. Analogy can also be used to prove one point based on the acceptance of another. For example, scientists found consistent distributions of Burkitt lym-phoma, falciparum malaria, and yellow fever in the tropics of Africa, and then they found the cause of Burkitt lymphoma (Burkitt lymphoma is a form of non-Hodgkin's lymphoma in which cancer starts in immune cells called B-cells). Through the method of analogy, it may be determined, if the patients with falciparum malaria are infected with yellow fever, Bur-kitt lymphoma may occur.

7.4　Causal Criteria

Strictly speaking, causal inference includes two aspects. One is whether a causal rela-tionship exists between events, which is the inference of qualitative conclusion. The second aspect is the strength of the causal relationship, and this is relatively more difficult to deter-mine. Causal inference should be based on corresponding criteria.

7.4.1　Causal Association

Association (also termed correlation, [statistical] dependence, relationship) refers to the statistical dependence between two or more events, characteristics, or other variables.

An association is present if the probability of the occurrence of an event or characteristic, or the quantity of a variable, depends upon the occurrence of one or more other events, the presence of one or more other characteristics, or the quantity of one or more other variables. The association between two variables is described as positive when higher values of a variable are associated with higher values of another variable. In a negative association, the occurrence of higher values of one variable is associated with lower values of the other variable. Associations can be broadly grouped under two headings, symmetrical or non-causal (see below) and asymmetrical or causal.

7.4.1.1 Asymmetrical Association

The definitive conditions of asymmetrical associations are direction and time. Independent variable X must cause changes in dependent variable Y; the "causal" variable must precede its "effect". The presence of certain criteria increase the likelihood of a true causal relationship, but the only essential criterion is that the cause must precede the effect.

①Direct association: directly associated, i. e. , not via a known third variable: A→B, referring only to causality.

②Indirect association, two types are distinguished: As shown in Figure 7. 7a, Factor C is associated with Disease A only because both are related to a common underlying Factor B. Alteration of Factor C will not produce an alteration in the frequency of Disease A un-

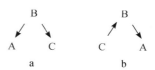

Figure 7. 7   Two Types of Indirect Association

less an alteration in C affects B. It has been suggested that to avoid confusion with the alternative meaning of indirect association, this type should be called "secondary association". In Figure 7. 7b, Factor C is associated with Disease A by means of an intermediate or intervening Factor B. Alteration of Factor C would produce an alteration in the frequency of Disease A. To avoid confusion, this type should be called "indirect causal association".

③Spurious association: A term, preferably avoided, used with different meanings by different authors. Spurious association may refer to artifactual, fortuitous, false secondary, or to all kinds of non-causal associations due to chance, bias, failure to control for extraneous variables, confounding, etc.

7.4.1.2 Symmetrical Association

An association is non-causal if it is symmetrical, as in the statement F = MA (force equals mass times acceleration). This is a non-causal, non-directional expression of the mathematical relationship between the physical properties of force, mass, and velocity. If one side of the equation changes, then the other must also change to maintain equilibrium.

Although epidemiologists are usually most interested in asymmetrical statements that have direction, the symmetrical equation can be useful. For instance, prevalence can be expressed in terms of incidence and duration in the simple approximation. P = I * D. If two of these three elements are known, the third can be derived.

　　To be specific, causal inference is the term used for working out whether observed associations are likely to be causal. Causal inference should not be made until certain requirements have been satisfied. These requirements fall under two major questions: ①Is there actually an association? ②If an association is present, is it likely to be causal?

　　We can determine association between the exposure and disease by formulating a "test hypothesis". Once we have identified an association, several steps must be addressed before we can declare causality. Figure 7. 8 gives the process of causal inference. We must rule out the interference of chance and all kinds of bias, and identify that exposure precedes the disease. Then, we can declare the causal-association by Hill's criteria. Specifically, the process is followed:

　　①The association is actually present and is statistically meaningful by the statistical test that rules out the interference of chance (random error).

　　②The association is not spurious (false). The spurious association, also called non-causal association, is attributed to the selection bias, information or measurement bias, and confounding bias.

　　③The confirmatory criteria for causality are satisfied. Even if a statistical association does not exist and is not due to bias, causal inference cannot be made confidently without satisfying the confirmatory criteria of causality. (The criteria are shown below.)

　　④Indirect association and direct association. The term "indirect association" may be used in a broader sense. An indirect causal association is inferred when the risk factor or independent variable causes changes in the dependent variable or condition through the mediation of other intermediate variables or conditions.

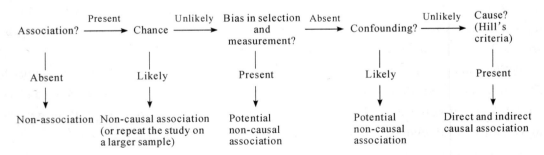

Figure 7. 8　The Process of Causal Inference

7.4.2　Hill's Criteria

　　After establishing a statistical association and ruling out sources of bias (system error), other specific criteria should be satisfied to support the causal inference. No absolute criteria will determine whether the observed association is a real causal association. In practice, lists of causal criteria have become popular, possibly because they seem to provide a road map through the complicated territory, and perhaps because they suggest hypotheses to be evaluated in a given problem. The causal criteria were stated by the various persons or agents, as shown in Table 7.1.

Table 7.1   The Causal Criteria Stated by Different Persons or Agents

Provider	Year	Number	Criteria
US Surgeon General's first report "Smoking and Health"	1964	5	a) Temporality b) Strength c) Specificity d) Consistency or repeatability e) Coherence
Hill	1965	8	Add 3 terms to the above criteria: a) Biologic gradient b) Biologic plausibility c) Experimental evidence
Su Delong	1980	8	Similar to Hill's criteria: a) Combination of consistency and plausibility b) Add to "consistency of distribution"
Lilienfeld	1994	7	Similar to Hill's criteria: a) Combination of consistency and plausibility

A commonly used set of criteria was based on a list of considerations proposed by Sir Austin Bradford Hill (1965). Hill's criteria expanded upon a list offered previously in the landmark US Surgeon General's first report "Smoking and Health". Hill emphasized that causal inferences cannot be based on a set of rules, condemned emphasis on statistical significance testing, and recognized the importance of many other factors in decision making.

These criteria serve as a general guide and are not meant to be a rigid list. Not all criteria must be fulfiled to establish scientific causation.

7.4.2.1   Temporality

Temporality refers to the necessity that the cause or risk factor C precedes the effect or disease D in time. This criterion is inarguable. Only if it is found that C cannot precede D, can we dispense with the causal hypothesis that C could cause D.

Of course, observations in which C precedes D may provide no evidence for or against the hypothesis that C can cause D in some instances. For example, the cock crowed, then the dawn came. It is important to pay attention to the time interval from cause to disease in chronic disease studies. Obviously, the disease cannot be attributed to asbestos if one person exposed to asbestos for three years developed lung cancer.

Among epidemiologic study designs, temporal relationship is shown more clearly in the experimental and cohort studies than in the case-control and cross-sectional studies.

7.4.2.2   Strength

The strength of association in epidemiologic studies is measured by the size of the effect, expressed as relative risk or relative rate (RR) or odds ratio (OR)(Table 7.2). The stronger the association, the more likely the causal relationship. Some suggest that RR > 3 in cohort studies, or OR > 4 in case-control studies, provides strong support for causation.

Table 7.2 The Range of RR and Its Significance

RR	Significance
0—0.3	Highly useful
0.4—0.5	Moderately useful
0.6—0.8	Vaguely useful
0.9—1.1	No impact
1.2—1.6	Vaguely harmful
1.7—3.0	Moderately harmful
>3.0	Highly hazardous

Not all strong associations are causal. Sometimes a strong association may be entirely or partially due to unmeasured confounders or other sources of modest bias. Of course, once the confounding factor is identified, the association is diminished by controlling for the factor. We can deduce this confounding factor is the cause. For example, a strong relation between Down syndrome and birth order was observed, which is confounded by maternal age.

Cornfield et al. (1959) acknowledged that a weak association does not rule out a causal connection. Today, some associations, such as those between smoking and cardiovascular disease or between environmental tobacco smoke and lung cancer, are accepted by most as causal even though the associations are considered weak. A strong association is neither necessary nor sufficient for causality, and a weak association is neither necessary nor sufficient for the absence of causality.

7.4.2.3 Consistency

Consistency refers to the repeated observation of an association in different populations under different circumstances. Causality is more likely when the association is supported by repeated observations. For example, more than 100 studies over the last 40 years demonstrated that smoking can increase the risk of lung cancer.

Lack of consistency, however, does not rule out a causal association, because some causes produce effects only under unusual circumstances. Blood transfusions can cause infection with human immunodeficiency virus (HIV), but they do not always do so: the virus must also be present. Consistency may only be apparent when all the relevant details of a causal mechanism are understood, which is very seldom.

7.4.2.4 Biologic Gradient

Biologic gradient refers to the presence of a dose-response or exposure-response curve with an expected shape. As the dose of exposure increases, the risk of disease occurrence also increases or decreases. For example, more smoking means more carcinogen exposure and more tissue damage, hence more opportunity for carcinogenesis. In a word, people who smoke the most cigarettes are more likely to suffer from lung cancer. In the cases of phocomelia, the condition varied in different regions and years according to the sales volume of thalidomide.

Associations that do show a monotonic trend in disease frequency with increasing levels of exposure are not necessarily causal. Confounding can result in a monotonic relation between a non-causal risk factor and disease if the confounding factor itself demonstrates a biologic gradient in its relationship with disease. The relationship between birth rank and Down syndrome shows a strong biologic gradient that merely reflects the progressive relation between maternal age and the occurrence of Down syndrome. A clear dose-response relationship (if present) can increase the likelihood of a causal association, although the absence of a dose-response relationship does not necessarily rule out a causal relationship.

7.4.2.5 Plausibility

Plausibility refers to the scientific likelihood of an association. The starting point is an epidemiologic association. To determine if an epidemiologic association is causal, one must consider its plausibility. Plausibility refers to consistency with what is known about a particular disease, including biological knowledge, prior beliefs, or knowledge. The causal relationship between hyperlipidemia and coronary heart disease (CHD) can be supported by pathological evidence of coronary atherosclerosis and animal experimental results.

7.4.2.6 Coherence

The term *coherence* implies that a causal association should not conflict with a disease's natural history and biology.

Hill's examples for coherence, such as the histopathologic effect of smoking on bronchial epithelium (in reference to the association between smoking and lung cancer) or the difference in lung cancer incidence by sex, could reasonably be considered examples of plausibility, as well as coherence; the distinction appears to be a narrow one.

Absence of coherence cannot be taken as evidence against causality. The presence of conflicting information may indeed refute a hypothesis, but one must always remember that conflicting information may be an error or a misinterpretation. An example is the "inhalation anomaly" in smoking and lung cancer, which is the fact that most lung cancers among smokers seem to be concentrated at sites in the upper airways of the lung. Several observers interpreted this anomaly as evidence that cigarettes were not responsible for the majority of cases. However, other observations suggested that cigarette-borne carcinogens were deposited preferentially where most lung cancer cases were observed, and so the anomaly was, in fact, consistent with a causal role for cigarettes (Wald, 1985).

In some books, coherence is interpreted as the consistency of distribution. The determinants of distribution should be consistent with geographical and other distributions of disease.

7.4.2.7   Experimental Evidence

Three types of experimental proof can be established: ①experiments in human subjects using the risk factor, which is seldom available; ②experiments in animals, which may not be relevant to human beings, and ③cessation effects of exposure.

Experimental evidence refers to "experimental or semi-experimental" evidence obtained from reducing or eliminating a putatively harmful exposure and seeing if the frequency of disease subsequently declines. Hill called this the strongest possible evidence of causality. It can be faulty, however, as the "semi-experimental" approach can be confounded or otherwise biased by a host of concomitant secular changes. Moreover, even if eliminating the exposure does causally reduce the frequency of disease, it might not be for the etiologic reason hypothesized. The draining of a swamp near a city, for instance, would predictably and causally reduce the rate of yellow fever or malaria in that city the following summer. But it would be a mistake to call this observation the strongest possible evidence of a causal role of miasmas (Poole, 1999).

7.4.2.8   Specificity

Specificity is: ①that a cause leads to a single effect, not multiple effects, and ②that an effect has one cause, not multiple causes. Specificity indicates that a single exposure is associated with only one disease.

Specificity strengthens the evidence for causality, but lack of specificity does not rule out causality. For example, the association between smoking and lung cancer is not specific because the causal factor of lung cancer is not merely smoking. However, we cannot deny the causality between the smoking and the lung cancer because of the existence of other evidence.

7.4.2.9   Analogy

Analogy isn't one of Hill's criteria. It has been suggested that, if the exposure/disease association is like other established causal associations, the case for causation is strengthened. But the absence of such analogies only reflects a lack of imagination or experience, not the falsity of the hypothesis.

(Sun Guixiang, Yao Meixue, Jenny Bowman, Zhao Jinshun)

Exercise

Chapter 8   Diagnostic Test

Accurate diagnosis is crucial to the clinical practice. With the rapid development of modern medical sciences and molecular biology techniques, the discovery of new diagnostic tests has been accelerated over the past few decades. How to assess the accuracy and value of new diagnostic tests? How about the clinical application and extended value? Can these new diagnostic tests replace the existing diagnostic methods? In order to solve such problems, we have to know how to assess the accuracy, reliability and clinical value of new diagnostic tests.

8.1   Introduction

8.1.1   Definition of Diagnostic Test

A diagnostic test is any kind of medical test performed to aid in the diagnosis or detection of disease. The commonly used diagnostic tests include physical examination, laboratory measurements, radiological imaging, clinical scores derived from questionnaires, and operative findings. Some of the diagnostic tests are parts of a simple physical examination which require only simple tools in the hands of a skilled practitioner and can be performed in an office environment. Other tests require elaborate equipment used by medical technologists or the use of a sterile operating theater environment. Some tests require samples of tissue or body fluids being delivered to a pathology lab for further analysis. Some simple chemical tests, such as urine pH, can be measured directly in the doctor's office. Most diagnostic tests are conducted on the living patients; however, some of these tests can also be carried out on a dead case as part of an autopsy. The primary purpose of diagnostic tests is to provide clinical information which can discriminate among disease states, thereby improving the physician's management of the patients.

8.1.2   Definition of Screening Test

A tenet of public health is that primary prevention of disease is the best approach. However, If all cases of disease cannot be prevented, then the next strategty is the early detection of disease in asymptomatic, apparently healthy individuals. Screening is defined as the presumptive identification of unrecongnized disease or defects by the application of tests, examinations, or other procedures that can be applied rapidly.

Screening is a strategy used in a population to identify an unrecognized disease in individuals without signs or symptoms. This can include individuals with pre-symptomatic or unrecognized symptomatic disease. As such, screening tests are somewhat unique in that they are performed on persons apparently in good health. Figure 8.1, a schematic representation of the course of the disease over time, illustrates the possibility of detecting the presence of disease earlier using a screening test, thereby allowing for more effective treatment and prolonged survival. There are two important concepts in this diagram: ①a screening test can identify individuals with a disease before the presence of disease is detected by routine diagnosis (e. g. , when symptoms occur), and ②treatment at the time of detection by screening, as opposed to the time of routine diagnosis, results in an improved outcome.

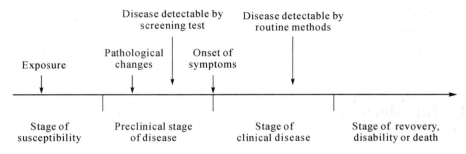

Figure 8.1　Natural History of a Disease over Time

Screening interventions are designed for early identification of disease in a community setting, thus enabling earlier intervention and management in the hope to reduce mortality and increase the quality of life. Although screening may lead to an earlier diagnosis, not all screening tests have been shown to benefit the person being screened. Over-diagnosis, misdiagnosis, and creating a false sense of security are potential adverse effects of screening. For these reasons, a test used in a screening program, especially for a disease with low incidence, must have good sensitivity in addition to acceptable specificity.

8.1.3　Screening Tests Versus Diagnostic Tests

Screening tests are not diagnostic tests. The primary purpose of screening tests is to identify early disease or risk factors for disease in large numbers of apparently healthy individuals. The purpose of diagnostic tests is to establish the presence (or absence) of a disease as a basis for treatment decision on people with symptoms or positive screening results (confirmatory test). Some of the key differences between screening tests and diagnostic tests are listed in Table 8.1.

Table 8. 1   Differences Between Screening Tests and Diagnostic Tests

Item	Diagnostic Tests	Screening Tests
Target population	Symptomatic individuals to establish a diagnosis or asymptomatic individuals with a positive screening test	Large numbers of asymptomatic, but potentially at-risk individuals
Purpose	To establish the presence/absence of a disease	To detect potential disease indicators
Test method	Maybe invasive, expensive but justifiable as necessary to establish the diagnosis	Simple and acceptable
Positive result threshold	Chosen toward high specificity. More weight is given to accuracy and precision than to patient acceptability	Generally chosen toward high sensitivity not to miss potential disease
Positive result	Result provides a definite diagnosis	Essentially indicates suspicion of a disease that warrants confirmation
Cost	Higher costs associated with diagnostic test may be justified to establish the diagnosis	Low cost, benefits should justify the costs since large numbers of people will need to be screened to identify a small number of potential cases

8. 2   Design of a Diagnostic Test

In this section, several aspects of a diagnostic test design are discussed, including the gold standard, selection of study subjects, determination of sample size and assessment form of results.

8. 2. 1   Gold Standard

The gold standard is the criterion by which it is decided that the patient has, or does not have, the disease. It is the best available test that is universally recognized by the clinical medical circles. Typical gold standards might be: a single diagnostic test that is known to be accurate, e. g. , contrast venography for deep vein thrombosis; a combination of diagnostic tests that will reliably rule in and rule out diseases (e. g. , lung perfusion scanning for pulmonary embolus combined with pulmonary angiography in equivocal cases); diagnostic testing with follow-up for negative cases to identify cases of disease that may have initially been misclassified as healthy. In most cases, gold standard is absolutely accurate, that is to say, it stands for truth. Because it is usually more expensive and more dangerous to use these more accurate ways of establishing the truth, clinicians and patients prefer simpler tests to the rigorous gold standard, at least initially. For example, chest x-rays and sputum smears are used to determine the nature of pneumonia, rather than lung biopsy with an examination of the diseased lung tissue.

An ideal gold standard should correctly classify patients with and without the disease.

It should also be safe and simple to apply because it would be unethical to ask patients to undergo dangerous or complex testing purely for research purposes. If an ideal gold standard does exist, then there is little need to evaluate new diagnostic tests.

8.2.2　Selection of Study Subjects

The study subjects should be representative of the population who would receive the test in routine practice. The diagnostic test evaluations assemble the study population by selecting patients on the basis of their gold standard test, selecting a group of patients with the disease (cases) and a group of people without the specific disease (controls).

8.2.2.1　Selection of Cases

Case identification should be complete, and the source of population from which cases arise should be well defined. Cases should be sampled at random from an appropriate spectrum of patients, who have been confirmed with the gold standard test. The representation of cases will directly affect the value of a diagnostic test.

8.2.2.2　Selection of Controls

Controls should be patients without the target disease, including the disease that used to be confused with the target ones, as the control group need the value of clinical differential diagnosis. Healthy persons are generally not included in the control group.

8.2.3　Determination of Sample Size

Determination of sample size for a diagnostic test is affected by various factors, including the sensitivity, specificity of the diagnostic test to be evaluated, significance level (α), and the allowable error (δ). Adequate sample size is necessary to guarantee the accuracy of the diagnostic test. The sample size might be determined by using a calculation formula or consulting relative sample size table. If both the sensitivity and specificity of a diagnostic test are evaluated close to 50%, then the sample size would be calculated as follows:

$$n=\left(\frac{u_a}{\delta}\right)^2 p(1-p)$$

n—the number of patients in the study; u—value for the cumulative probability equal to $\alpha/2$; δ—allowable error; p—the estimation of sensitivity and specificity for a diagnostic test (sensitivity for cases, specificity for controls)

If both the sensitivity and specificity of a diagnostic test are evaluated to be less than 20% or greater than 80%, then the sample size would be calculated as follows:

$$n=[57.3u_a/\arcsin(\delta/\sqrt{p(1-p)})]^2$$

8.2.4　Assessment Form

To evaluate the diagnostic test, it is necessary to establish a definite way to decide if someone has a particular condition. For example, to diagnose cancer, you could take a biopsy; to diagnose the depression, you could look for key symptoms in a psychiatry consultation; to diagnose a walking problem, you could video a patient and have it viewed by an expert. This is called the "gold standard" but is usually expensive and difficult to administer. We may require a diagnostic test which is cheaper and easier to use. Initially, we will consider a simple binary situation in which both the gold standard and the novel diagnostic test have either a positive or negative outcome (disease is present or absent). The situation is best summarized by the following table (Table 8. 2). In writing this table, we should always put the gold standard on top and the results of the novel diagnostic test on the side. Any diagnostic test can be evaluated in this manner. The first step in the evaluation of a diagnostic test is to determine the true status of the disease. In the whole procedure, the gold standard is considered to represent the true status of the disease.

Table 8. 2   Standard Table for a Novel Diagnostic Test

Novel	Gold Standard		Diagnostic Test
	Positive	Negative	
Positive	a True positive	b False positive	$a+b$
Negative	c False negative	d True negative	$c+d$
Total	$a+c$	$b+d$	$n=a+b+c+d$

a—the numbers of true positive (diagnosed positive who do have the condition).
b—the numbers of false positive (diagnosed positive who do not have the condition).
c—the numbers of false negative (although the test is negative, the subjects do have the disease).
d—the numbers of true negative (diagnosed negative who do not have the condition).

8.3   Evaluation of a Diagnostic Test

A diagnostic test can be evaluated in the form of Table 8. 2.

8.3.1   Terms for Evaluating Diagnostic Tests

The following terms are often used to evaluate the diagnostic test. It is well worth being sure that you know exactly what they mean. Specificity, in particular, is often confused with positive predictive value (PV+).

8.3.1.1   Sensitivity (Se)

Sensitivity relates to the test's ability to identify positive results. The sensitivity of a test refers to the ability of the test to correctly identify patients with the disease. It is also known as true positive rate. Sensitivity is calculated as follows:

$$S_p = \frac{a}{a+c} \times 100\%$$

The greater the sensitivity of a test is, the more likely the test will detect persons with the disease of interest. A test with high sensitivity can be considered as a reliable indicator when its result is negative since it rarely misses true positives among those who are actually positive. For example, a sensitivity of 100% means that the test recognizes all actual positives. Thus, in contrast to a high specificity test, negative results in a high sensitivity test are used to rule out the disease. That is, a negative result would virtually exclude the possibility that the patient has the disease of interest. A test with high sensitivity has a low type II error rate.

8.3.1.2　Specificity (Sp)

Specificity relates to the test's ability to identify negative results. The specificity of a test is defined as the proportion of patients that are known not to have the disease who will test negative for it. Specificity is calculated as follows:

$$\text{Sp} = \frac{d}{b+d} \times 100\%$$

The greater the specificity of a test is, the more likely the person without the disease of interest will be excluded from the consideration of having the disease. Tests with high specificity are often used to confirm the presence of a disease. Highly specific tests rarely miss negative outcomes so they can be considered reliable when the result is positive. Therefore, a positive result from a test with high specificity means a high probability of the presence of disease. A test with high specificity has a low type I error rate.

Sensitivity and specificity are descriptors of the accuracy of the diagnostic test. They are useful when deciding whether to perform the test. Depending on the clinical scenario, high sensitivity or specificity may be more important and the best test can be chosen for the clinical situation. If 100 patients known to have a disease were tested and 43 were positive, then the test had a 43% sensitivity. If 100 persons without disease were tested and 96 returned negative results, the test had a 96% specificity. Sensitivity and specificity are prevalence-independent test characteristics, as their values are intrinsic to the test and do not depend on the disease prevalence in the population of interest.

It is obviously desirable to have a test with both high sensitivity and high specificity. Unfortunately, it is usually not possible in practice. Instead, there is a trade-off between the sensitivity and specificity of a diagnostic test. This is true whenever clinical data takes on a range of values. In those situations, the location of a cut-off point, the point on the continuum between normal and abnormal, is an arbitrary decision. As a consequence, for any given test result expressed on a continuous scale, one characteristic (e. g. , sensitivity) can be increased at the expense of the other (e. g. , specificity). Table 8.3 demonstrates this interrelationship for the diagnosis of diabetes. If we take 180mg/100ml as a cut-off point to diagnose diabetes, all of the people diagnosed as "diabetic" would certainly have the disease, but many other people with diabetes would be missed using this extremely demanding definition of the disease. The test would be very specific at the expense of sensitivity. At the other extreme, if anyone with a blood glucose lever >70mg/100ml was diagnosed as diabetic, very few people with the disease would be missed, but most normal people would be falsely labeled as having diabetes. The test would then be sensitive but nonspecific. There is no way, using a single blood sugar determination under standard conditions, that one can improve both the sensitivity and specificity of the test at the same time.

Table 8. 3　Trade-off Between Sensitivity and Specificity When Diagnosing Diabetes

Blood Sugar Level (2 hrs. after eating) (mg/100ml)	Sensitivity (%)	Specificity (%)
70	98. 6	8. 8
80	97. 1	25. 5
90	94. 3	47. 6
100	88. 6	69. 8
110	85. 7	84. 1
120	71. 4	92. 5
130	64. 3	96. 9
140	57. 1	99. 4
150	50. 0	99. 6
160	47. 1	99. 8
170	42. 9	100. 0
180	38. 6	100. 0
190	34. 3	100. 0
200	27. 1	100. 0

Source: Adapted from Public Health Service. *Diabetes Program Guide*. Washington, D. C. : US Government Printing Office, 1960

8. 3. 1. 3　False Negative (FN) Rate

The false negative rate, also known as the omission diagnostic rate, is defined as the percentage of persons with the disease of interest who have negative test results. The false negative rate is calculated as follows:

$$FN=\frac{c}{a+c}\times100\%=1-Se$$

8. 3. 1. 4　False Positive (FP) Rate

The false positive rate, also known as the misdiagnosis rate, is defined as the percentage of persons without the disease of interest who have positive test results. False positive rate is calculated as follows:

$$FP=\frac{b}{b+d}\times100\%=1-Sp$$

8. 3. 1. 5　Predictive Value

Two measures concerning the estimation of the probability of the presence or absence of disease are the positive predictive value (PV+) and the negative predictive value (PV−).

①The PV+ is defined as the percentage of persons with positive test results who actually have the disease of interest. The PV+ therefore allows us to estimate how likely it is that the disease of interest is present if the test is positive. The PV+ is calculated as follows:

$$PV+ = \frac{a}{a+b} \times 100\%$$

②The PV− is defined as the percentage of persons with negative test results who do not have the disease of interest. The general formula for the calculation of PV−is:

$$PV- = \frac{d}{b+d} \times 100\%$$

If the prevalence, sensitivity, and specificity are known, the positive predictive value can be obtained from the following identity:

$$PV+ = \frac{P \times Se}{P \times Se + (1-P) \times (1-Sp)} \times 100\%$$

Similarly, the negative predictive value can be obtained from the following identity:

$$PV- = \frac{(1-P) \times Sp}{(1-P) \times Sp + P \times (1-Se)} \times 100\%$$

Positive and negative predictive values measure the usefulness of a result once the test has been performed. For example, a PV+ of 80% indicates that 80% of patients with a positive test result truly have the disease. A PV− of 40% indicates that only 40% of patients testing negative are truly healthy. Prevalence is also called prior probability, the probability of disease before the test result is known. PV+ and PV− are influenced values by the prevalence of the disease in the population that is being tested.

The predictive value of a test is not a property of the test alone. It is determined by the sensitivity and specificity of the test and the prevalence of the disease in the population being tested. The more sensitive a test is, the higher the negative predictive value will be (the clinician can be more confident that a negative test result rules out the disease being sought). Conversely, the more specific the test is, the better its positive predictive value will be (the more confident the clinician can be that a positive test confirms or rules in the diagnosis being sought). Because predictive value is also influenced by prevalence, it is not independent of the setting in which the test is used. Positive results even for a very specific test, when being applied to patients with a low likelihood of having the disease, will be largely false positives. Similarly, negative results, even for a very sensitive test, when being applied to patients with a high chance of having the disease, are likely to be false negatives. In sum, the interpretation of a positive or negative diagnostic test result varies from setting to setting, according to the estimated prevalence of the disease in a particular population.

It is not intuitively obvious what prevalence has to do with an individual patient. For those who are skeptical it might help to consider how a test would perform at the extremes of prevalence. No matter how sensitive and specific a test might be, there will be a small proportion of patients who are misclassified by it. Imagine a population has no case of the disease. In such a group, all positive results, even for a very specific test, will be false positives. Therefore, if the prevalence of the disease in a population approaches zero, the positive predictive value of a test also approaches zero. If the prevalence approaches 100%, the negative predictive value approaches zero.

8. 3. 1. 6   Likelihood Ratios

Another set of measures is useful in the interpretation of diagnostic tests. The likelihood ratios (LR) provide a more useful way of presenting diagnostic data and can be applied to individual patients in a way that sensitivity and specificity cannot be. The LR is the probability of a particular test result for a person with the disease of interest divided by the probability of that test result for a person without the disease of interest. Two versions of the likelihood ratio exist and they are known as the likelihood ratio for a positive test result (LR +) and likelihood ratio for a negative test result (LR—).

①The likelihood ratio for a positive test result is the probability of a positive test result for a person with the disease of interest divided by the probability of a positive test result for a person without the disease. Mathematically, the LR+ is calculated as:

$$LR+ = \frac{Se}{1-Sp} = \left[\frac{a/(a+c)}{b/(b+d)} \right]$$

In the above formula, sensitivity and specificity are expressed as proportions rather than as percentages. The smallest possible value of the LR+ occurs when the numerator is minimized (Se=0), producing an LR+ of zero. The maximum value of the LR+ occurs when the denominator is minimized (Sp=1, so 1−Sp=0), resulting in an LR+ of positive infinity. An LR+ of one indicates a test with no value in sorting out persons with and without the disease of interest since the probability of a positive test result is equal for affected and unaffected persons. Values of the LR+ greater than one corresponds to situations in which persons affected with the disease of interest are more likely to have a positive test result than unaffected persons. The larger the value of the LR+ is, the stronger the association between having a positive test result and having the disease of interest is.

②The likelihood ratio for a negative test result is the probability of a negative test result for a person with the disease of interest divided by the probability of a negative test result for a person without the disease. Mathematically, the LR— is calculated as:

$$LR- = \frac{1-Se}{Sp} = \left[\frac{c/(a+c)}{d/(b+d)} \right]$$

In the above formula, sensitivity and specificity are also expressed as proportions rather than as percentages. The smallest possible value of the LR— occurs when the numerator is minimized (Se=1, so 1−Se=0), producing an LR— of zero. The maximum value of the LR— occurs when the denominator is minimized (Sp=0), resulting in an LR— of positive infinity. An LR— of one indicates a test with no value in sorting out persons with and without the disease of interest, since the probability of a negative test result is equally likely for affected and unaffected persons. The smaller the value of the LR— is, the stronger the association between having a negative test result and not having the disease of interest is.

One of the desirable properties of the likelihood ratios is that they do not vary as a function of the prevalence of the disease. That is to say, in contrast to a predictive value, the likelihood ratios do not vary according to the prevalence of the disease. As indicated above, these two likelihood ratios indicate the strength of the linkage between a test result and the likelihood of disease. A diagnostic test with a large LR+ value increases the suspicion of disease for patients with positive test results. The larger the size of the LR+ is, the better the diagnostic value of the test will be. An LR+ value of 10 or greater is often considered as an indication of a test of high diagnostic value.

Similar reasoning applies to LR−, except in the opposite direction. A diagnostic test with a small LR− value decreases the suspicion of disease for patients with negative test results. The smaller the size of the LR− is, the better the diagnostic value of the test will be. An LR− value of 0.1 or less is often considered as an indication of a test of high diagnostic value.

8.3.1.7　Agreement Rate

A diagnostic test or clinical finding is unreliable if it gives different results when being performed by different clinicians. For example, if two radiologists frequently produce conflicting reports from the same computed tomography (CT) scan, then CT scanning (in this circumstance) is an unreliable test. Evaluations of diagnostic tests should include some assessment of reliability. The agreement rate can be a descriptor of the reliability and can be calculated as follows:

$$\text{Agreement Rate} = \frac{a+d}{a+b+c+d} \times 100\%$$

8.3.1.8　Kappa Value

In fact, reliability cannot be estimated by simply measuring the percentage agreement between two observers because the agreement may occur simply by chance. For example, if a test has only two possible results (positive and negative) then there is a 50% probability that two observers will agree in their interpretation purely by chance.

The most common method for estimating reliability is to measure the kappa score. This calculates the agreement between observers beyond that expected due to chance. Values range from −1 (completely opposite) to 1 (perfect agreement). The kappa score of 0 indicates an agreement by chance only. Values related to kappa are as follows (n refers to a total number of samples):

①Observed agreement (P_o): $P_o = \dfrac{a+d}{n} \times 100\%$;

②Agreement of chance (P_c): $P_c = \dfrac{[(a+b) \times (a+c)/n][(c+d) \times (b+d)/n]}{n}$;

③Potential agreement beyond chance$=1-P_c$;

④Actual agreement beyond chance$=P_o-P_c$;

⑤ $Kappa = \dfrac{P_o - P_c}{1 - P_c}.$

8.3.2   ROC Curves

In clinical medicine, classification data, especially dichotomous data is commonplace and useful. Examples of dichotomous results are a positive or negative history of pain in a breast, the presence or absence of a palpable breast mass on physical examination, and a normal or abnormal alkaline phosphatase level (a serum marker of bone or liver disease). In many situations, however, test results often occur in the form of continuous variables. Breast pain, for example, can be negative, intermittent, or continuous. The size of a breast mass is usually measured in centimeters. A serum alkaline phosphatase level may range along a continuous scale. Generally, the more extreme the value of a continuous test result is, the greater the likelihood that the result reflects a laboratory error or an abnormality in the patient.

Objects are often classified based on a continuous random variable. For example, if the blood protein levels in diseased people and healthy people are normally distributed with means of 2 g/dL and 1 g/dL, respectively, a medical test might measure the level of a certain protein in a blood sample and classify any number above a certain threshold as indicating disease. The experimenter can adjust the threshold (black vertical line in Figure 8.2, also known as the cutoff point), which will, in turn, change the false positive rate. Increasing the threshold would result in fewer false positives, more true negatives, fewer true positives, and more false negatives. Moving the cutoff point changes the test's sensitivity and specificity. A convenient summary of the above relationship can be shown in a graph referred to as a receiver operating characteristic (ROC) curve.

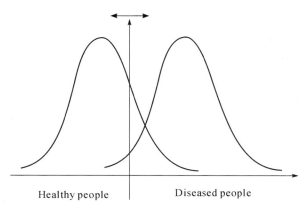

Figure 8.2   Distribution of Blood Protein Levels in Healthy People and Diseased People

ROC analysis is part of a field called "Signal Detection Theory" developed during World War II for the analysis of radar images. Radar operators had to decide whether a blip on the screen represented an enemy target, a friendly ship, or just noise. Signal detection theory measures the ability of radar receiver operators to make these important distinctions. Their ability to do so was called the "Receiver Operating Characteristics". In radiology, ROC analysis is a common technique to evaluate new radiology techniques. In social sciences, ROC analysis is often called the ROC Accuracy Ratio, a common technique for judging the accuracy of default probability models. ROC curves are also used extensively in epidemiology and medical research and are frequently mentioned in conjunction with evidence-based medicine. In medicine, ROC analysis has been extensively used in the evaluation of diagnostic tests.

To draw ROC curves, only the true positive rate and false positive rate are needed (as functions of some classifier parameter). The true positive rate defines how many correct positive results occur among all positive samples available during the test. False positive rate, on the other hand, defines how many incorrect positive results occur among all negative samples available during the test. The ROC space is defined by false positive rate and true positive rate as x and y-axes respectively, which depicts relative trade-offs between true positive (benefits) and false positive (costs). Since the true positive rate is equivalent with sensitivity and the false positive rate is equal to 1—specificity, the ROC graph is sometimes called the sensitivity vs. (1—specificity) plot. At each cutoff point, sensitivity and 1—specificity will be calculated. These results then can be graphed along with the full range of cutoff points, producing the ROC curve.

A hypothetical example of ROC curves is shown in Figure 8. 3. In the graph, the performance of the diagnostic test is shown by the solid line. A completely random guess would give a point along the dashed diagonal line (the so-called line of no-discrimination) from the left bottom to the top right corners. An intuitive example of random guessing is a decision by flipping coins (heads or tails). At every point along the dashed line, the sensitivity is equal to 1—specificity. As the size of the sample increases, a random classifier's ROC point migrates toward (0.5, 0.5). When the sensitivity is equal to 1—specificity, the numerator of the LR+ is equal to its denominator. That is to say, at every point along the dashed diagonal line the LR+ is equal to one, and a positive test result is equally likely for persons with and without the disease interest. A diagnostic test that is clinically useful, therefore, will have the ROC curve that is far from the dashed diagonal line.

The best possible prediction method would yield a point in coordinate (0, 1) or the upper left corner of the ROC space, representing 100% sensitivity (no false negatives) and 100% specificity (no false positives). The (0, 1) point is also called a perfect classification. The choice of the particular cut-off value for a test is essentially a decision informed by the attempt to maximize sensitivity and specificity. Generally, there is a trade-off between sensitivity and specificity, and the decision must be based on their relative importance. However, the decision to use a diagnostic test depends not only on the ROC analysis but also on the ultimate benefit to the patient. The prevalence of the outcome, which is the pre-test probability, must also be known.

A summary index of overall test performance can be calculated as the area under the

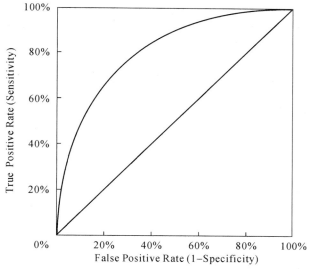

Figure 8.3   A Hypothetical Example of ROC Curves

ROC curve (AUC). The greater the area is, the better the test performance will be. The highest possible value for the area under a ROC curve is 1, which is equivalent to a perfect test. In contrast, the area under the dashed diagonal line, corresponding to a test that does not distinguish between persons with and without the disease of interest, is 0.5. An AUC of 0.5 indicates that a test based on that variable would be equally likely to produce false positive or true positive results. This principle also can be used to compare the overall performance of multiple hypothetical diagnostic tests for a particular condition. Figure 8.4 shows an example of ROC curves for both lactate and urea as markers for predicting the risk of death. The area under the ROC curve is greater for test urea than for test lactate, suggesting that urea is a better diagnostic test than lactate.

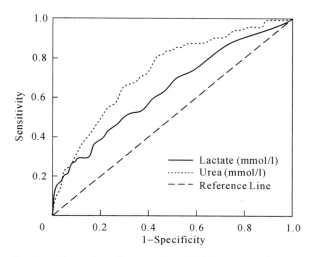

Figure 8.4   Receiver Operating Characteristic (ROC) Curves for Lactate and Urea

Source: Adapted from Bewick (1960)

8. 4   Improving the Efficiency of a Diagnostic Test

8. 4. 1   Choosing the Population with a High Prevalence Rate

When the sensitivity and specificity of diagnostic tests remain constant, the prevalence rate is proportional to the positive predictive value. In the case of constant property of the diagnostic test, as the prevalence increases, the positive predictive value increases. Thus, diagnostic tests which are carried out in the high-risk populations have high positive predictive value. In clinical practice, if the prevalence rate of a population is 40% — 60%, the diagnostic test could well confirm or exclude cases. Therefore, it is suggested to conduct the diagnostic test in the population with a high prevalence rate.

8. 4. 2   Combination of Tests

In clinical practice, clinicians always want to find a diagnostic test with both high sensitivity and specificity. However, there are few, if any, such diagnostic tests. It is difficult to confirm diagnosis only relying on a certain diagnostic test. To improve the efficiency of a diagnostic test, multiple tests are combined together. A combination of tests is routinely used in many diagnostic studies, with the most commonly adopted schemes, parallel and serial interpretation (Table 8. 4).

Parallel interpretation schemes, also known as "OR" schemes, are used to increase sensitivity. Serial interpretations schemes, also known as "AND" schemes, are used when the goal is to increase the specificity of diagnosis. Serial interpretation is commonly used when the cost of a false-positive diagnosis is high.

Table 8. 4   Combination of Tests

Combination of Tests	Test A	Test B	Total Result
Parallel Test	+	+	+
	+	−	+
	−	+	+
	−	−	−
Serial Test	+	+	+
	+	−	−
	−	+	−
	−	−	−

8.4.2.1   Parallel Tests

Parallel tests are also known as the "OR" scheme, in which the disease diagnosis is considered positive given any positive value observed in any test applied. Generally, the sensitivity of a diagnostic test is overestimated in the parallel test, and the negative predictive value for a given disease is higher than each individual test used. On the contrary, specificity and positive predictive value are underestimated. In other words, the disease is less likely to be missed, but false-positive results are prone to occur in the parallel test. The degree to which sensitivity and negative predictive value increase depending on the extent to which the tests identify patients with the disease missed by the other tests used. Given the individual sensitivity for Test A and Test B is SE_A and SE_B respectively, while the specificity is indicated as SP_A and SP_B, the calculation of the sensitivity and specificity for parallel testing are as follows:

$$\text{Sensitivity of parallel test} = SE_A + SE_B \times (1 + SE_A)$$
$$\text{Specificity of parallel test} = SP_A \times SP_B$$

For example, given that two diagnostic tests used in a parallel test have a sensitivity of 60% and 80% respectively, the sensitivity of the parallel test will be only 80% if the cases detected by a test with 60% sensitivity are completely overlapped by another test with 80% of sensitivity. If the detection of disease by two tests can make up for each other, the sensitivity will undoubtedly be 100%. If the two tests are completely independent of each other, the sensitivity of parallel testing will be 92%.

Parallel testing is particularly useful when the clinician is in need of a sensitive test but has available only two or more relatively insensitive ones that measure different clinician phenomena. By using the tests in parallel, the net effect is a more sensitive diagnostic strategy. However, the parallel test increases the risk of treating healthy (false positive) patients.

8.4.2.2   Serial Tests

Serial tests are also known as "AND" schemes, in which all individual test must obtain a positive result in order to make a "positive diagnosis". Physicians most commonly use serial testing strategies in clinical situations where the rapid assessment of patients is not required, such as in office practices and hospital clinics in which ambulatory patients are followed over time. Serial testing is also used when some of the tests are expensive or risky and is only applied when simpler and safer tests suggest a diagnosis of disease. Serial testing leads to less laboratory use than parallel testing because additional evaluation is contingent on prior test results. However, the serial tests usually take more time because additional tests are ordered only after the results of previous ones become available.

Serial testing maximizes specificity and positive predictive value but reduces sensitivity and negative predictive value. One ends up more definitive that positive test results represent disease, but runs an increased risk that disease will be missed. Serial testing is particularly useful when none of the individual tests is highly specific.

    In case of a physician is going to use two tests in series, the process will be more efficient if the test with the highest specificity is used first. For example, Test A is more specific than Test B, whereas Test B is more sensitive than Test A. By using Test A firstly, fewer patients are subjected to both tests, even though equal numbers of diseased patients are diagnosed, regardless of the sequence of tests. However, if one test is much cheaper or less risky, it may be more prudent to use it at first. The sensitivity and the specificity of serial testing are calculated respectively as follows:

$$\text{Sensitivity of serial test} = SE_A \times SE_B$$
$$\text{Specificity of serial test} = SP_A + SP_B \times (1 - SP_A)$$

Example: A total of 7,840 patients with myocardial infarction are diagnosed by serum enzyme Test A and serum enzyme Test B, respectively. The test results are shown in table 8.5. The Se, Sp, PV(+) and PV(−) of parallel tests and serial tests respectively are shown below.

Table 8.5   The Result of Serum Enzyme Test A and Serum Enzyme Test B

Test Results		Patient Group	Non-Patient Group
Test A	Test B		
+	−	14	10
−	+	33	11
+	+	117	21
−	−	35	7599
Total		199	7641

Source: Adapted from Wang Jianhua (2003)

Parallel test:

Se = (14+33+117)/199 × 100% = 82.41%

Sp = 7599/7641 × 100% = 99.45%

PV+ = (14+33+117)/(14+33+117+10+11+21) × 100% = 79.61%

PV− = 7599/(7599+35) × 100% = 99.54%

Serial test:

Se = 117/199 × 100% = 58.79%

Sp = (10+11+7599)/7641 × 100% = 99.73%

PV+ = 117/(117+21) × 100% = 84.78%

PV− = (10+11+7599)/(10+11+7599+14+33+35) × 100% = 98.94%

8.5   Bias

Both diagnostic tests and screening tests are important components of modern medical care. However, many of them are not rigorously evaluated before general application. Studies examining test characteristics often have methodological flaws that impair their ability to provide reliable information on test performance. These flaws can introduce systematic nonrandom errors (biases) that distort measures of test accuracy. Other errors can make it difficult to generalize the results of individual studies. These problems may enhance the apparent performance of poor tests while obscuring the performance of good tests, and they may result in the widespread use of tests with uncertain of limited efficacy.

8.5.1   Bias in Diagnostic Tests

8.5.1.1   Verification Bias

Verification bias occurs when a study is restricted to patients who have definitive verification of disease. It is one type of measurement bias, in which the results of a diagnostic test affect whether the gold standard procedure is used to verify the test result. This type of bias is also known as "work-up bias" or "referral bias". In clinical practice, referral bias is more likely to occur when a preliminary diagnostic test is negative. Because many gold standard tests can be invasive, expensive, and carry high risk (e. g. , angiography, biopsy, surgery), patients and physicians may be more reluctant to undergo a further workup if a preliminary test is negative. In cohort studies, obtaining a gold standard test on every patient may not always be ethical, practical, or cost effective. These studies can thus be subjected to verification bias. In most situations, verification bias introduces an overestimated sensitivity but an underestimated specificity.

In the case of positive test results, patients selected for an additional workup are more likely to have the disease than those excluded and therefore are more likely to have a true-positive result. Alternatively, patients with negative results may truly have a disease that goes undetected because definitive testing was not performed. These cases would normally increase the number of false-negative reports. However, as these cases are not identified they are falsely labeled as true negatives. In general, workup bias related to positive diagnostic tests leads to underdiagnosis of the disease, but not the overdiagnosis. This leads to high estimates of both sensitivity and negative predictive value. One method to reduce verification bias in clinical studies is to perform gold standard testing in a random sample of study participants.

8.5.1.2   Spectrum Bias

Spectrum bias refers to the phenomenon that the performance of a diagnostic test may vary in different clinical settings due to different patient populations, which lead to low generalization of test performance. These differences are interpreted as spectrum bias. This type of bias is also known as "subgroup bias" or "case-mix bias". Mathematically, the spectrum bias is a sampling bias but different from traditional statistical bias. This has led some authors to refer to the phenomenon as spectrum effects, whilst others maintain it as bias if the true performance of the test differs from that which is "expected". Usually, the performance of a diagnostic test is measured in terms of its sensitivity and specificity and it is changed when referring to spectrum bias. However, other performance measures such as the likelihood ratios may also be affected by spectrum bias.

Generally, spectrum bias could be caused by three reasons. The first is due to a change in the case-mix of those patients with the target disorder (disease) and this affects the sensitivity. The second is due to a change in the case-mix of those without the target disorder (disease-free) and this affects the specificity. The third is due to a change in the prevalence, and this affects both the sensitivity and specificity. The third reason is not widely appreciated, but there is plenty of empirical evidence suggesting that it does indeed affect a test's performance. Examples where the sensitivity and specificity change between different subgroups of patients may be found with the carcinoembryonic antigen test and urinary dipstick tests.

Diagnostic test performances reported by some studies might be artificially overestimated in case-control study design, in which a healthy population ("fittest of the fit") is compared with a population with the disease ("sickest of the sick"). That is two extreme populations are compared, rather than typical healthy and diseased populations.

If properly analyzed, recognition of the heterogeneity of subgroups can lead to insights about the test's performance in varying populations.

8.5.2　Bias in Screening Tests

8.5.2.1　Lead Time Bias

Lead time is the length of time between the detection of disease (usually based on new, experimental criteria) and its clinical presentation and diagnosis (based on traditional criteria). Lead time bias occurs when two diagnostic tests are compared, and one test (the screening test) diagnoses the disease earlier, but there is no effect on the outcome of the disease—it may appear that the test prolonged survival, when in fact it only results in earlier diagnosis compared to traditional methods. It is an important factor when evaluating the effectiveness of a specific test.

As shown in Figure 8.5, the person detected with or without screening dies at the same time, but the time from diagnosis until death is greater for the screened patient because the cancer was recognized at an earlier point in time. The time from early diagnosis by screening to routine diagnosis is defined as the lead time.

The aim of screening is to diagnose a disease at an early stage. Without screening, the disease might be discovered at an advanced stage. Even though the patient will die at the same time because the disease was diagnosed early with screening, the survival time since diagnosis is longer for patient detected by screening. No additional life has been gained (and indeed, there may be added anxiety as the patient must live with the knowledge of the disease for longer). For example, most patients with Huntington's disease are diagnosed when symptoms appear around the age of 50 years, who will die around at the age of 65 years. Most patients, therefore, survive about 15 years after the diagnosis. With a genetic test, it is possible to diagnose this disorder at birth. If this newborn baby dies around age 65, he or she will have "survived" 65 years after the diagnosis, without having lived any longer than the people who were diagnosed late in life.

According to raw statistics, screening seems to increase survival time (the gained time is called lead time). If we do not think about what survival time actually means in this context, we might attribute success to a screening test that does nothing but advance diagnosis. Lead time bias can affect the interpretation of the survival rate.

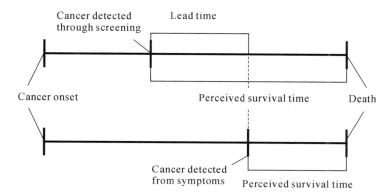

Figure 8.5   A Comparison of a Patient with a Routine Clinical Diagnosis of Disease and a Patient with Disease Detected by Screening

8.5.2.2   Length Time Bias

Length time bias is a form of selection bias, a statistical distortion of results which can lead to incorrect conclusions about the data. Length time bias can occur when the lengths of intervals are analyzed by selecting intervals that occupy randomly chosen points in time or space. This process favors longer intervals, thus skewing the data.

Length time bias is often discussed in the context of the benefits of cancer screening, where it can lead to the perception that screening leads to better outcomes when it has no effect. Fast-growing tumors generally have a shorter asymptomatic phase than slower-growing tumors. This means that there is a shorter period when the cancer is present in the body (and therefore might be detected by screening) but not yet large enough to cause symptoms, which would cause the patient to seek medical care and be diagnosed without screening. As a result, if the same number of slow-growing and fast-growing tumors appear in a year, the screening test will detect more slow-growers than fast-growers. If these slow-growing tumors are less likely to be fatal than the fast growers are, the people whose cancer is detected by screening will do better, on average, than the people whose tumors are detected from symptoms (or at autopsy), even if there is no real benefit to detect cancer earlier. The impression is that detecting cancers through screening causes cancers to be less dangerous when the reality is that less dangerous cancers are simply more likely to be detected by screening.

(Li Xiaofeng, Lin Yulan, Wong Li Ping, Zhao Jinshun)

Exercise

Chapter 9　Communicable Disease Epidemiology

Communicable diseases constituted the most serious health issue in the world until the beginning of the 20th century when chronic diseases began to dominate this scenario in developed countries. The terminology and concepts used today in the epidemiology of communicable diseases evolve from a complex set of scientific fields that studied their agents, causes and determinants, dynamics of transmission and diffusion of these agents, and means of prevention. Many of these concepts were established throughout the 19th century and at the beginning of the 20th century.

9.1　Introduction

9.1.1　Definition and Characteristics of Communicable Diseases

Communicable diseases, or infectious diseases, are caused by the presence of microbes and can be transmitted to humans from other humans, animals or the environment. These kinds of diseases are also called transmissible diseases due to the potential of transmission from one person to another. To define a given disease as a communicable disease, Koch's postulates (first proposed by Robert Koch) must be satisfied:

①The microorganism must be found in abundance in all organisms suffering from the disease, but should not be found in healthy organisms.

②The microorganism must be isolated from a diseased organism and grown in pure culture.

③The cultured microorganism can cause the disease when it is introduced into a healthy organism.

④The microorganism can be isolated from the inoculated, diseased experimental host and identified as being identical to the original specific causative agent.

However, not all criteria could be met during the identification of a new infectious disease. There are healthy carriers with asymptomatic infections who can still transmit the disease to others. In other cases, the causative agent cannot be isolated. For example, *Treponema pallidum*, the causative agent of syphilis, cannot be cultured in vitro; however, the organism can be cultured in rabbit testes.

9.1.2　The Burden of Communicable Diseases

Table 9.1 showed the incidence of selected infectious diseases in 2004 based on the data of WHO. Diarrheal disease affected far more individuals than any other illness (including noncommunicable diseases), even in high-income countries. Pneumonia and other lower respiratory tract infections were the second most common cause of illness globally, in all regions except Africa.

Table 9. 1　Incidence of Selected Infectious Diseases by WHO Region, 2004 (Millions)

	World	Africa	The Americas	Eastern Mediterranean	Europe	South-East Asia	Western Pacific
Tuberculosis[a]	7. 8	1. 4	0. 4	0. 6	0. 6	2. 8	2. 1
HIV infection[a]	2. 8	1. 9	0. 2	0. 1	0. 2	0. 2	0. 1
Diarrhoeal Disease[b]	4620. 4	912. 9	543. 1	424. 9	207. 1	1276. 5	1255. 9
Pertussis[b]	18. 4	5. 2	1. 2	1. 6	0. 7	7. 5	2. 1
Measles[a]	27. 1	5. 3	0. 0[c]	1. 0	0. 2	17. 4	3. 3
Tetanus[b]	0. 3	0. 1	0. 0	0. 1	0. 0	0. 1	0. 0
Meningitis[b]	0. 7	0. 3	0. 1	0. 1	0. 0	0. 2	0. 1
Malaria[b]	241. 3	203. 9	2. 9	8. 6	0. 0	23. 3	2. 7
Dengue[b]	9. 0	0. 1	1. 4	0. 5	0. 0	4. 6	2. 3
Lower Respiratory Infections[b]	429. 2	131. 3	45. 4	52. 7	19. 0	134. 6	46. 2

[a] new cases; [b] episodes of illness; [c] An entry of 0. 0 in the table refers to an incidence of less than 0. 05 million (less than 50,000); Source: Adapted from WHO (2008)

During 2000 to 2011, lower respiratory infections, diarrhea and HIV/AIDS have remained the top major killers. Lower respiratory infections caused 3. 2 million deaths in 2011, only behind the line of ischemic heart disease and stroke. Global HIV/AIDS deaths are projected to rise from 2. 2 million in 2008 to a maximum of 2. 4 million in 2012. Tuberculosis is no longer among the top 10 leading causes of death, but is still among the top 15, killing one million people in 2011.

Infectious diseases pose a significant threat in low-income countries. Lower respiratory infections, HIV/AIDS, diarrheal diseases, malaria and tuberculosis collectively account for almost one-third of all deaths in these countries (Figure 9. 1).

Children under 5 years old are highly susceptible to infections. In 2011, 6. 9 million children died before reaching their fifth birthday; almost all (99%) of these deaths occurred in low- and middle-income countries. The major killers of children aged less than 5 were pneumonia, prematurity, birth asphyxia and birth trauma, and diarrheal diseases. Malaria was still a major cause of death in sub-Saharan Africa, causing about 14% of under-five deaths in the region.

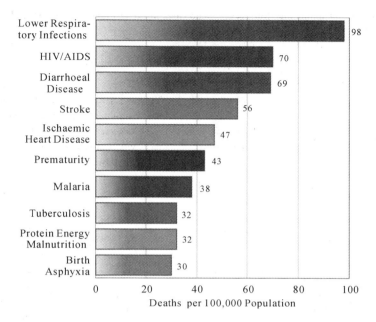

Figure 9. 1   Top 10 Causes of Death in Low-Income Countries, 2011
Source: Adapted from WHO (2008)

9. 1. 3   New and Reemerging Infectious Diseases

"Emerging" infections are defined to have newly appeared in the population or have existed but rapidly increasing in an incidence or geographic range. The concepts of emerging diseases and disease emergence were used as a practical approach to focus attention and research on new pathogens and disease evolution in a changing world.

There are three types of emerging infectious diseases:

①Emergence of an unedited infectious disease (an unknown newly described pathogen, a new clinical picture, and a known pathogen).

②Reemergence, after a prolonged period of silence, of a previously known infectious disease.

③Spread of a known infectious disease among new territories and/or virgin populations.

Specific factors are responsible for disease emergence and they can be identified in virtually all case studies.

Table 9. 2 listed major emerging infectious diseases and the factors responsible for emergence since 1973.

Table 9. 2   Domains and Emergence Conditions of Some Emerging Infectious Diseases

Year of Emergence	Emerging Disease	Pathogenic Agent	Place and Domain of Emergence	Factors of Emergence	
				Main Probable Factor	Secondary Factor
1983	AIDS	HIV	US; urban communities	Yet nor entirely understood origin of the virus introduction; sexual contact with or exposure to blood or tissues of an infected person	Changes in lifestyles; increasing international travel; multiple sexual partners; increased intravenous drug addiction; vertical transmission; invasive medical technology
1986	Bovine spongiform encephalopathy in cows	Prion	Great Britain; cattle rising area	Feeding cattle with products containing prion infected sheep tissue	Changes in the rendering process
1986	Human monocytic erlichiosis	Ehrlichia chaffeensis	US	Unknown; tick is suspected vector	Increased recognition; possibly increase in host and vector populations
1993	Hantavirus pulmonary syndrome	Sin Nombre virus (Hantavirus)	US, " four corners" area	Human invasion of virus ecologic niche by rice field agriculture; close contact with the infected rodent natural reservoir; inhalation of aerosolized rodent urine and feces	Climatic condition favoring a rodent pullulation
1997	Highly pathogenic avian influenza	H5N1 influenza virus	Hong Kong; chicken farms of Southeast Asia	Animal-animal influenza virus reassortment; emergence H5N1 avian influenza virus reassortant; extensive chicken farming	Integrated pig-duck agriculture; close contact with infected chicken
2003	Severe acute respiratory syndrome	SARS coronavirus	South province of China	Eating practices of infected wild animals (viverrids)	Catching and preparing infected Civetta
2005	Chikungunya arthritis	Chikungunya virus	Indian Ocean Islands	Introduction of the virus in the islands (Comore, Reunion) by a yet to be discovered mean (plane, wind?)	Pullulation of infected competent mosquito, lack of control

Source: Adapted from Tibayrenc (2007)

9. 1. 4 Factors Impact on Infectious Disease

9. 1. 4. 1 Changes in Human Demographics and Behavior

Human population movements or upheavals, caused by migration or war, are important factors in disease emergence. In many parts of the world, economic conditions are encouraging the mass movement of workers from rural areas to urban cities. The newly introduced infection would have the opportunity to spread along highways and by airplane. The frequency of the most severe form, dengue hemorrhagic fever, which is thought to occur when a person is sequentially infected by two types of dengue virus, is increasing as different dengue viruses have extended their range and now overlap.

Human behavior can affect disease dissemination. The best-known example is sexually transmitted disease. Human behavior as sex or intravenous drug use have contributed to the emergence of HIV are now well known. Motivating appropriate individual behavior and constructive action will be essential for controlling emerging infections. However, human behavior remains one of the weakest links in disease control and places a big challenge for all scientists.

9. 1. 4. 2 International Travel and Commerce

In the past, an infection introduced into people in a geographically isolated area might be brought to a new place through travel, commerce, or war. Trade between Asia and Europe, perhaps beginning with the silk route and continuing with Crusades, brought the rat and bubonic plague to Europe. Beginning in the 16th and 17th centuries, ships bringing slaves from West Africa to the New World also brought yellow fever and its mosquito vector to the new territories. In the 19th century, cholera had similar chance to spread from its probable origin in the Ganges plain to the Middle East and, from there, to Europe and much of the remaining world. Each of these infections had once been localized and took advantage of opportunities to be carried to previously unfamiliar parts of the world. Today, opportunities have become far richer and more numerous, reflecting the increasing volume, scope, and speed of traffic in an increasingly mobile world. The Asian tiger mosquito was introduced into the United States, Brazil, and parts of Africa in shipments of used tires from Asia. Since its introduction in 1982, this mosquito has established itself in at least 18 states of the United States and has acquired local virus including Eastern equine encephalomyelitis, a cause of serious disease. Another mosquito-borne disease, malaria, is one of the most frequently imported diseases in nonendemic areas, and cases of airport malaria are occasionally identified.

9. 1. 4. 3 Technology and Industry Development

Modern production methods yield increased efficiency and reduced costs but can increase the chances of contamination and amplify the effects of such contamination. The problem is further compounded by globalization. A pathogen present in the raw material may find its way into a large batch of the final product, as happened with the contamination of hamburg-er meat by *E. coli* O157. Bovine spongiform encephalopathy (BSE), which emerged in Great Britain, was likely an interspecies transfer of scrapie from sheep to cattle. That occurred when changes in rendering processes led to incomplete inactivation of scrapie agent in sheep byproducts fed to cattle.

Medical products are also at the front line of exposure to new diseases. In the outbreak of Ebola fever in Africa, many of the secondary cases were hospital-acquired, most transmit-ted to other patients through contaminated hypodermic apparatus, and some to the health care staff by contact.

Advance in microbiology and medicine can also lead to the new recognition of agents that are already widespread. A good example is the bacterium *Helicobacter pylori*, a proba-ble cause of gastric ulcers and some cancers. We have lived with these diseases for a long time without knowing the cause. Recognition of the agent is often advantageous, offering a new promise of controlling a previously intractable disease, such as treating gastric ulcers with antimicrobial therapy.

9.1.4.4 Microbial Adaption and Change

The emergence of antibiotic-resistant bacteria is an evolutionary lesson on microbial ad-aptation, as well as a demonstration of the power of natural selection. Selection for antibiot-ic-resistant bacteria and drug-resistant parasites has become frequent, driven by inappropri-ate use of antimicrobial drugs in a variety of applications. Pathogens can also acquire resist-ance genes from other species in the environment. The evolution of a new variant may result in a new expression of disease. The epidemic of Brazilian purpuric fever in 1990, associated with a newly emerged clonal variant of *Hemophilus influenza*, is an example.

9.1.4.5 Breakdown of Public Health System and Infrastructure

Classical public health and sanitation measures have long served to minimize dissemina-tion and human exposure to many pathogens spread by traditional routes such as water or preventable by immunization or vector control. Breakdowns in preventive measures may lead to disasters. Cholera, for example, has been raging in South America and Africa in this cen-tury. The rapid spread of cholera in South America may have been abetted by reductions in chlorine levels used to treat water supplies. The success of cholera and other enteric diseases is often due to the lack of a reliable water supply. The outbreak of waterborne *Cryptospo-ridium* infection in Wisconsin, the United States, in the spring of 1993, with over 400,000 estimated cases, was in part due to a nonfunctioning water filtration plant.

9.1.5 Roles of the Epidemiology of Communicable Diseases

The modern epidemiological approach to communicable diseases focuses on the interac-tion of the disease agent, the host and the environment. Epidemiology gives us tools to learn about how these factors interact to produce a disease in a population. A complete understanding of the causative agent and transmission is always useful but not necessary. The most famous example is that of John Snow and the London cholera epidemic of 1854.

Unlike the epidemiology of non-communicable diseases, there are some unique principles of communicable disease epidemiology.

①Studies of communicable disease epidemiology usually involve two or more populations:

- Humans;
- Infectious agents—bacteria, fungi, viruses, helminths, etc. ;
- Vectors—mosquitoes, snails, ticks, mites, etc. ;
- Animals—dogs, mice, sheep, bats, etc.

②Infection in one person can be transmitted to others, and thus a case is also a risk factor.

③The cause of communicable disease is often known. An infectious agent is a necessary cause. Epidemiology studies are then used for:

- Identification of causes of new, emerging infections, e. g. , HIV, SARS;
- Surveillance of communicable diseases;
- Identification of the source of outbreaks;
- Studies of routes of transmission and natural history of infections;
- Identification of new interventions.

9.2 Etiology of Communicable Diseases

The epidemiologic triad is a good model to investigate the etiology of communicable diseases (Figure 9. 2). Based on that model, the disease is the result of forces within a dynamic system consisting of agent of infection, host, and environment.

①Agent: microorganisms adapt to changing conditions, including human control efforts such as antibiotics.

②Host: human populations are constantly growing and moving as people age, travel, and migrate into a new environment.

③Environment: changes occur locally and globally, both naturally and through human intervention.

Each disease is influenced by a set of factors. Some foodborne diseases, such as salmonella, are highly dependent on environmental factors such as cross-contamination and cooking/holding temperatures. The spread of measles is influenced by immunization status, but also by housing conditions and nutritional status. Disease history is a big factor with some diseases, such as hepatitis A, which confer lifetime immunity after infection. Many other diseases can cause repeated infections in the same individual, for example, gonorrhea, shigellosis and malaria. Some diseases are transmitted to humans only through arthropod vectors such as mosquitoes, ticks or lice.

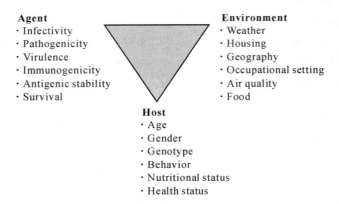

Figure 9. 2   Epidemiology Triad of Communicable Diseases

9. 2. 1   Biological Characteristics of Agents

Microorganisms have multiple strategies to enable continued growth in a hostile environment. The mechanism behind pathogenesis is complex. Some biological characteristics of microbes are important in understanding the pathogenesis of infection (Table 9. 3).

9. 2. 1. 1   Infectivity

It is the ability of a pathogen to get colonized inside a host body. The infectivity is evaluated by the percentage of the infected subjects among the susceptible contactors, which is also called a secondary attack rate.

9. 2. 1. 2   Pathogenicity

It is the ability of a pathogen to cause illness in a host. The pathogenicity is evaluated by the number of the subjects with clinical symptoms divided by the number of infected subjects.

9. 2. 1. 3   Virulence

It is the ability of a pathogen to cause the severe outcome of the disease. The virulence is evaluated by the percentage of the deaths in the diseased ones.

9. 2. 1. 4   Variability

It includes antigen variation, virulence variation, drug resistance variation and parasite host variation.

Table 9. 3   Ranking of Infection by Infectivity, Pathogenicity, and Virulence

Severity*	Infectivity	Pathogenicity	Virulence
High	Smallpox measles chickenpox	Smallpox rabies measles chickenpox common cold	Rabies smallpox tuberculosis leprosy
Intermediate	Rubella mumps common cold	Rubella mumps	Poliomyelitis measles
Low	Tuberculosis	Poliomyelitis tuberculosis	Measles chickenpox
Very low	Leprosy	Leprosy	Rubella common cold

* The "severity" of infection varies by how it is being measured.

Source: Adapted from Nelson (2007)

9. 2. 2   Host

A person who provides hospitality for pathogens is called a host. Animals and plants can also be hosts of the pathogens which cause diseases in their species. When we are talking about human disease, animals are called vectors of pathogens. Some diseases can be transmitted from animals to humans. In that case, the diseases are then called zoonosis-borne diseases as well as anthropozoonosis. Susceptible hosts provide the possibility for the occurrence and dissemination of communicable diseases.

Host (human) factors are closely related to the epidemic of infectious diseases which mainly include age, sex, race, genetic factors, physiological function, nutritional status, previous infection history, and behavior patterns, etc.

9. 2. 3   Environment

Many environmental factors may inhibit or promote disease transmission and hence influence the epidemic process of communicable diseases. Natural factors and social factors all play a role, of which social factors are particularly important.

9. 2. 3. 1   Natural Factors

Natural factors include climate, geography, soil, animals and plants, etc. Climate and geography are the most significant factors. Many infectious diseases show local and seasonal characteristics, which are mainly related to the influence of climate and geographical factors on animal infectious sources. For example, the incidence rate of brucellosis is higher in spring because spring is the peak period of litter and abortion of animals (sheep, cattle, etc.) and the lactation period. Insect-borne infectious diseases are most obviously affected by natural factors. The geographical distribution, seasonal growth and decline, activity ability of vector organisms and the development and reproduction of pathogens in vector organisms are all restricted by natural factors, thus affecting the epidemic characteristics of infectious diseases. For example, the high incidence of dengue fever in summer and autumn is related to the breeding of Aedes mosquitoes. With global warming, the mosquito activity season is prolonged and the activity area is expanded. The virus proliferates actively in mosquitoes, and the pathogenicity and virulence of dengue virus are enhanced; the epidemic range of dengue fever expands from tropical and subtropical regions to temperate regions, and the epidemic intensity increases. Natural factors can change the epidemic characteristics of infectious diseases by affecting human life habits and body resistance. For example, in the hot summer weather, people eat more raw and cold food, increasing the chance of intestinal infectious diseases.

9.2.3.2 Social Factors

Social factors include human activities, such as production and living conditions, health habits, medical and health conditions, living environment, population mobility, lifestyles, customs, religious beliefs, social unrest and social systems. Compared with natural factors, social factors have a greater influence on the epidemic process of infectious diseases. In recent years, the prevalence of new and recurrent infectious diseases has been greatly influenced by social factors. Production and living conditions have an obvious influence on infectious diseases. For example, people who work barefoot in paddy fields or catch shrimps by fishing are vulnerable to schistosomiasis. Herdsmen who give birth to ewes suffering from brucellosis are prone to brucellosis. Congestion and poor indoor sanitation facilities can all lead to the spread of respiratory and intestinal infectious diseases. Malnutrition is associated with the occurrence of many infectious diseases. Lifestyles, customs, religious beliefs and other factors can also affect the popular process. For example, drug abuse, prostitution and men having sex with men have led to an increase in the incidence of sexually transmitted diseases. Medical and health conditions play an important role in infectious diseases. For example, in areas where immunization programs are well implemented, the incidence and mortality rates of poliomyelitis, measles, tuberculosis, whooping cough, diphtheria and tetanus have decreased significantly. Population movements have accelerated the spread of infectious diseases. With the increase of international/domestic exchanges and tourism, infectious diseases such as yellow fever and dengue fever spread to other countries. Economic crisis, war or turmoil, refugee flows and other factors have promoted the spread of infectious diseases. For example, the abuse of antibiotics and insecticides has increased the drug resistance of pathogens and vectors. The government's emphasis on the prevention and control of infectious diseases directly affects the prevalence and spread of infectious diseases. For example, strict management of infectious sources can effectively control the spread of diseases.

9.3   Infectious Process and Spectrum of Communicable Diseases

9.3.1   Infectious Process

The microorganisms exist everywhere in our environment and there are many occasions on which the microbes encounter humans. However, infectious diseases are not happening so frequently. Some organisms can peacefully coexist with humans and others may cause infections. Whether a disease can happen or not lies like the interaction between pathogens and hosts. This infection process is a biological process comprising a series of stages including:

9.3.1.1   Acquisition

The initial point of contact with a given microbial species. Acquisition can be endogenous or exogenous, depending on the sources and routes of organisms acquired.

9.3.1.2   Colonization

To establish a biological niche in a new habitat. Acquisition of a new microbial species may result in nothing more than a brief encounter. Colonization requires the microorganisms to successfully compete against an established indigenous microbial flora and counter local defense mechanisms. Once survive and replicate on a body surface, an organism is said to have colonized that site.

9.3.1.3   Penetration

To break the surface barrier and get deep inside the host body. A breach may happen in the epithelium like surgical wounds, skin lesions, or insect bites. Some parasites can penetrate intact skin. Droplet nuclei less than 5μm diameter can reach the alveoli and cause infection of the respiratory system.

9.3.1.4   Spread

An invading microorganism may spread by one or more routes: extension through surrounding tissues, via blood circulation or lymphatic vessels. Spread via the vascular route is particularly effective to deliver organisms all around the body quickly. During the dissemination of pathogens, breaking down host defenses is very crucial.

9.3.1.5   Damage

The function of organs, tissues or cells may be altered or damaged following the microbial invasion. Such changes can be caused by either pathogen cells or toxins secreted. The inflammatory reaction can be taken as the sign of host response to against damage.

9.3.1.6   Resolution

Host immune responses include humoral or cell-mediated immune. These reactions may cause damage of invading microbes through swelling, increased fragility of tissues, the formation of pus, scarring or necrosis. Failure to clear out pathogens may lead to the latency of chronic intracellular infection.

9.3.2　Spectrum of Communicable Diseases

Many microorganisms have evolved the capacity to engage their hosts in complex intimate interactions aiming at securing replication and transmission to a new host rather than at causing diseases. The co-evolutionary process between pathogens and their hosts usually lead to a peaceful relationship. Sometimes, however, the pathogens cause damage to the hosts. In some instances, disease symptoms may be an unpleasant manifestation of a self-limiting process. Pathogens get the chance to transmit from one host to the next and their hosts acquire immunity through the process. In other cases, the fatal disease may occur when the delicate balance is broken by a relatively strong pathogen and a weakened host.

If many individuals are equally exposed to an infectious agent, there may be a broad range of responses (Figure 9.3):

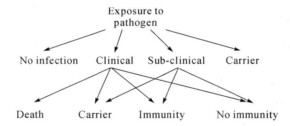

Figure 9.3　Variable Outcomes of Exposure to Pathogens

①Some do not become infected at all.
②Some become infected but develop no symptoms.
③Some become infected and develop mild or moderate symptoms.
④Some become infected and develop severe symptoms.
⑤Some die as a result of infection.

Each outcome accounts for a different proportion of total exposure to pathogens, and thus it is called the spectrum of infection or gradient of infection. The spectrum of disease presented in individuals ranges from subclinical infection to active cases. Briefly, there are three kinds of spectrums:

①The majority is a subclinical infection and severe cases are very rare. Hepatitis A, polio, and encephalitis B typically belong to this type.

②Most infected individuals show obvious symptoms and are easily diagnosed and treated. Severe cases are also rare. Common diseases include measles and chickenpox.

③Most infected individuals appear severe clinical symptoms and currently, there are no effective cures. For example, the morbidity of rabies is almost 100%.

Part of this variation is due to the capacity of the agent to produce disease. Infection of a healthy adult population with salmonella is likely to result in mostly unapparent or mild cases, with only a few people showing more severe symptoms and having very few deaths. On the other end of the spectrum, infections with rabies almost always result in severe illness and death.

Part of the variation is due to different levels of resistance of the hosts. If measles is introduced into a highly immunized population, then most individuals do not become infected. If measles is introduced into an unimmunized nutritionally deprived population, the spectrum shifts toward severe symptoms and may cause a high death rate.

The existence of the infectious disease spectrum can make it challenging to find out the extent of transmission in a specific population. For diseases with more subclinical infections, the infection spectrum often appears an iceberg shape (Figure 9. 4). The active clinical disease usually accounts for a relatively small proportion of the exposed or infected population. Fatal cases are analogous to the tip of an iceberg. Most unapparent infections hide underneath the ocean surface. The part of subclinically infected individuals has particularly epidemic importance because asymptomatic ones can still transmit the disease to other susceptible hosts. Isolation of potential carriers is difficult and screening for these carriers is highly necessary to control the dissemination of disease. If an infection has taken place, no matter in symptomatic or asymptomatic individuals, at least a 4-fold elevation of sera antibody should be observed. Therefore, backups of blood samples at the acute infection stage and recovery stage are recommended for a definite diagnosis.

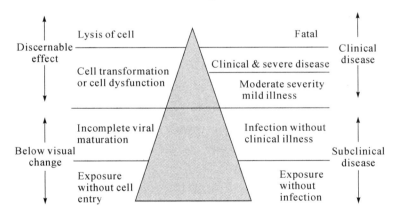

Figure 9. 4　Iceberg Phenomenon of Infectious Disease

9. 4　Three Links in the Epidemic Process

The epidemic process of communicable diseases is different from the infectious process and refers to the development and transmission of a disease in a population. This process can be concluded as Figure 9. 5. Microorganisms causing infectious diseases parasitize on the host and persist due to continuous reproduction of new generations. Living inside its host, the microorganism persists for a definite period. Then the pathogenic microorganism can survive by changing its residence, i. e. , by moving to another host via a corresponding transmission mechanism. This continuous chain of successive transmission of infection is called an epidemic process.

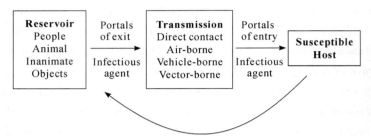

Figure 9. 5   Chain of Infection

An epidemic focus is the residence of infection source including the surrounding territory within the boundaries of which, the source can transmit a given disease through the pathogenic agent under given conditions. The focus of infection remains active until the pathogenic microorganisms are completely eradicated, plus the maximal incubation period in persons that were in contact with the source of infection.

There are three key links of the epidemic process: reservoir or source of infection, route of transmission, and susceptible population. These three obligatory factors are necessary for the onset and continuous course of an epidemic process.

9. 4. 1   Reservoirs

The reservoir is the usual habitat in which the agent lives and multiplies. Depending upon the agent, the reservoir may be humans, animals, and/or environment. Accordingly, infectious diseases are classed as anthroponoses (the source of infection is a man), zoonoses (the source of infection is animal), and anthropozoonoses (both man and animal can be the source of infection). When working with any disease agent, it is important to learn about its usual reservoir(s).

9. 4. 1. 1   Human Reservoirs

There are two types of human reservoirs, acute clinical cases and carriers.

①Acute clinical cases are people who are infected with the disease agent and become ill.

• Acute clinical cases are highly infectious due to high agent counts they possess and release.

• Because they are ill, their contacts and activities may be limited. They are also more likely to be diagnosed and treated than carriers are.

• Importance of a clinical case as a reservoir is determined by the quantity and frequency to discharge pathogens.

The danger of infection spreading from the patient depends on the period of the disease. During the incubation period, the role of the patient is not great because the pathogenic microorganism resides inside tissues and is seldom released. The pathogenic agents are released into the environment during the late incubation period only in measles, cholera, dysentery, and some other diseases. The greatest quantity of microbes is released during the advanced stage of the disease. This stage is usually associated with clinical manifestations of the disease such as frequent stools, vomiting, sneezing and cough.

②Carriers, on the other hand, are people who harbor infectious agents but are not ill.

• Carriers may present more risk for disease transmission than acute clinical cases because their contacts are unaware of the infection, and their activities are not restricted by illness.

• Importance of a carrier as a reservoir is determined by the quantity and frequency to discharge pathogens, as well as his/her social occupation.

• Depending on the disease, any of the following types of carriers may be important:

Incubatory carriers are people who are going to become ill but begin transmitting their infection before symptoms start. For example, a person infected with measles begins to shed the virus in nasal and throat secretions one or two days before the occurrence of any cold symptoms or rashes.

Unapparent infections. People with unapparent infections never develop an illness, but can transmit their infection to others. With some diseases, unapparent infections are more common than acute clinical cases. For example, among 100 individuals infected with the poliomyelitis virus, only one becomes paralyzed, and four will have mild illness with fever, malaise, headache, nausea and vomiting. But 95 out of the 100 will have no symptoms at all, although they pass the virus in their feces. Sometimes the likelihood of an unapparent infection depends on another epidemiological factor, such as age. Hepatitis A is a good example of this.

Subclinical infections. With some diseases, such as meningococcal meningitis, the number of subclinical cases may be quite high before a single clinical case appears. On some military bases where outbreaks have occurred, the carrier rate has been documented at 50% or more.

Convalescent carriers are people who continue to be infectious during and even after recovery from illness. This happens with many diseases. For example, salmonella patients may excrete the bacteria in feces for several weeks and occasionally for a year or more. This is more common in infants and young children. Treatment with inappropriate antibiotics may prolong the convalescent carrier phase.

Chronic carriers are people who continue to harbor infections for a long time after their recovery. For example, the chronic carrier state is common following hepatitis B infection, whether the person became ill or not, and may be lifelong. The risk of developing chronic hepatitis B depends on the person's age at infection. About 90% of infants being infected at birth become chronic carriers of the disease, compared with only 1-10% infected after age 5. Due to this reason, it is very important to give hepatitis B vaccine to newborns.

9.4.1.2 Animal Reservoirs

Animal reservoirs of infectious agents can be described in the same way as human reservoirs. They may be acute clinical cases or carriers. Parallel terms are referring to disease patterns in animals that may affect humans:

- Zoonosis—an infection or an infectious disease is transmissible under natural conditions between vertebrate animals and man;
  - Enzootic—"endemic" among animal populations;
  - Epizootic—"epidemic" among animal populations.

9.4.1.3 Environmental Reservoirs

Plants, soil and water may serve as the reservoir of infection for a variety of diseases. Most fungal agents (mycoses) live and multiply in soil. The organism that causes histoplasmosis lives in soil with high organic contents and undisturbed bird droppings. The agents that cause tetanus, anthrax and botulism are widely distributed in soil. The agent of Legionnaires' Disease lives in water, including water heaters.

9.4.2 Routes of Transmission

The combination of routes by which the pathogenic microorganisms are transmitted from an infected host to a healthy one is called the mechanism of infection transmission. Four mechanisms of infection transmission are distinguished according to the primary localization of pathogenic agents in hosts, including fecal-oral (intestinal localization), air-borne (airways localization), transmissive (localization in the blood circulating system), and contact (transmission of infection through direct contact with another person or environmental objects).

Three phases are distinguished in the transmission of infection from one host to another, including excretion from an infected host, presence in the environment, and ingress into a healthy host.

9.4.2.1 Direct Transmission

Many diseases are transmitted by direct contact with the human, animal or environmental reservoir. Prime examples are sexually transmitted diseases and enteric diseases such as shigella, giardia and campylobacter. Contact with soil may lead to mycotic (fungal) diseases. Droplet spread is also considered the direct transmission. Infectious aerosols produced by coughing or sneezing can transmit infection directly to susceptible people up to three feet away. Many respiratory diseases are spread this way.

9.4.2.2 Indirect Transmission

It may occur through animate or inanimate mechanisms.

① Animate mechanisms involve vectors, usually arthropods. These disease organisms may have complex life cycles that pass through several hosts. Flies may transmit infectious agents such as shigella in a purely mechanical way, by walking on feces and then on food.

Mosquitoes, ticks or fleas may serve as reservoirs for the growth and multiplication of agents, for example in malaria or Lyme disease. Vectors are subject to agents, hosts and environment factors too.

②Inanimate mechanisms: When disease agents are spread by environmental vehicles or by air, this is referred to as indirect transmission by inanimate mechanisms.

- Food is a common vehicle for salmonella infections.
- Water is the usual vehicle in cholera outbreaks.
- Surgical instruments and implanted medical devices may be the vehicles of staphylococcal infections.

Indirect airborne transmission is important in some respiratory diseases. This occurs when very tiny particles of respiratory material become suspended in the air (called aerosols). Such particles may remain suspended and stay infectious for varying periods. They are particularly dangerous because their size (1 to 5 microns) allows them to be drawn deep into the lungs and retained. Air may also spread particles of various sizes from contaminated soil, or objects such as clothing and floors.

9.4.2.3　Categories of Communicable Diseases by Routes of Transmission

(1)Air-Borne Diseases

Air is an important factor of direct transmission of respiratory infections. From the source of infection, microorganisms get into the air together with droplets of sputum. They are expelled in great quantities during sneezing, cough and conversation. Droplets of sputum containing the pathogenic microorganisms often remain suspended in the air for hours and can sometimes be carried from one enclosure to another with air streams and precipitate on environmental objects. After frying, sputum droplets infect dust which is then inhaled by a healthy person. Dust infection is feasible only with those microorganisms that persist in the environment and can survive in the absence of water.

Tuberculosis is spread primarily through exhaled or coughed droplets and is a significant cause of morbidity and mortality throughout the world. Other highly important diseases spread by person-to-person contact include influenza, measles, the common cold, and staphylococcal skin infections.

(2)Food-Borne Diseases

About 75% of the new infectious diseases affecting humans over the past 10 years were caused by bacteria, viruses and other pathogens that started in animals and animal products. Many of these diseases in people are related to the handling of infected domestic and wild animals during food production in food markets and at slaughterhouses. Food-borne diseases are caused when microbes, or their toxins, enter the body through the consumption of food or beverages. Milk and meat are common transmission media. Dairy products (curds, sour cream), vegetables, fruits, berries, bread and other foods that are not fully cooked before use are important transmission factors as well. Most cases of the food-borne disease are caused by bacteria or viruses, but parasites and prions, such as the one that causes variant

Creutzfeldt-Jakob encephalopathy, can also be spread through food. Food-borne diseases are believed to occur more frequently in developing countries, but outbreaks occur in both developing and industrialized countries and can affect large numbers of people. For instance, an outbreak of hepatitis A in China caused by the consumption of contaminated clams affected more than 300,000 individuals in 1988, and an outbreak of salmonellosis caused by the consumption of contaminated ice cream affected 224,000 people in the United States in 1994.

(3) Water-Borne Diseases

Water is another important medium by which infection can be transmitted. Pathogenic microorganisms can get into the water by various ways: with effluents, sewage, with runoff water, due to improper maintenance of wells, laundry, animal watering, getting of dead rodents into the water, etc. Water can be the medium for the transmission of cholera, typhoid fever, leptospirosis, dysentery, viral hepatitis A, and other diseases. Infections that result from contact with water-borne pathogens can result in either endemic or epidemic diseases. If potable water gets contaminated with fecal sewage, the water-borne infection can become epidemic with rapid spreading. The elderly and immunocompromised populations are also at an increased risk for water-borne infections.

Cholera is a spectacular example of water-borne disease. It is characterized as an acute enteric disease with sudden onset of copious watery diarrhea, vomiting, rapid dehydration, acidosis, and circulatory collapse. Caused by the bacterial agent *Vibrio cholerae*, it still occurs as acute epidemics in many parts of the developing world.

(4) Soil-Borne Diseases

Soil is contaminated by excrements of humans and animals, various wasters, dead humans and animals. Contamination of soil is an important epidemiologic factor because soil is the habitat and site of the multiplication of flies, rodents, etc. Eggs of some helminths (ascarids, *Trichuris trichiura*, hookworms) are incubated in soil. The pathogenic microorganisms of soil can pass into water, vegetables, fruits that are eaten by man. It is especially dangerous to use fecal sewage to fertilize soil where cucumbers, tomatoes and other vegetables are grown. Tetanus, gangrene, and anthrax are transmitted through soil.

(5) Blood-Borne Diseases

Blood-borne diseases are caused by pathogens such as viruses or bacteria that are carried in the blood. The most common blood-borne diseases are hepatitis B, hepatitis C, and HIV/AIDS. Outbreaks of hemorrhagic fevers and Ebola have occurred in Africa and other parts of the world since 1976. Common routes of infection with blood-borne diseases include unprotected sexual activity, contact with blood through needles or other sharps, and transmission from mother to child during delivery.

(6) Sexually Transmitted Diseases

Sexually transmitted diseases (STDs), also commonly referred to as sexually transmitted infections (STIs), are primarily spread through the exchange of body fluids during sexual contact. STDs may also be transmitted through blood-to-blood contact and from a woman to her baby during pregnancy or delivery (congenital transmission). Exposure to STDs can occur through any close exposure to the genitals, rectums, or mouths. Unprotected sexual contact increases the likelihood of contracting an STD. Abstaining from sexual contact can prevent STDs, and correct and consistent use of latex condoms reduces the risk of transmission.

(7)Vector-Borne Diseases

Vector-borne diseases are caused by bacteria, viruses, or parasites that are transmitted to humans by animal vectors. Vectors can be divided into two groups: specific and non-specific (mechanical). Specific carriers such as lice, fleas, and mosquitoes transmit infection by sucking blood (inoculation) or contaminating human skin with their excrement. Inside specific transmitters of infection, the pathogenic microorganisms multiply, accumulate, and with time become dangerous to the surrounding. Non-specific carriers transmit the pathogenic microorganisms by a pure mechanical method. Flies, for example, carry microbes of dysentery, typhoid fever, viral hepatitis and some other diseases that are found on their bodily surfaces, on the limbs, in the proboscis, and the intestine.

Vector-borne diseases are most common in tropical and subtropical regions where optimal temperatures and moisture levels promote the reproduction of arthropods, especially mosquitoes. Diseases such as malaria, dengue, sleeping sickness, and arthropod-borne encephalitis have occurred and, in some instances, are still present at endemic or epidemic levels. Re-emergence of vector-borne disease is a constant concern due to the rapid rate at which they are capable of spreading. The response to these diseases has played a large role in integrating public health agencies, research, and relief and assistance to areas that are troubled by vector-borne pathogens.

(8)Zoonotic Diseases

Infectious diseases of humans can be divided into those that are communicable only between humans and those that are communicable to humans from nonhuman vertebrate animals (those with backbones such as mammals, birds, reptiles, amphibians, and fish). Infectious diseases that have vertebrate reservoirs and are potentially transmissible to humans under natural conditions are called the zoonosis. Examples are rabies and plague. Zoonotic diseases may be either enzootic (like endemic in human diseases) or epizootic (like an epidemic in human diseases). Because of the large number of domestic and wild animals that can serve as a source of zoonotic diseases and the numerous means of transmission, zoonotic diseases are often difficult to control. Public health veterinarians have a critical role in zoonotic disease surveillance, prevention and control, but risk reduction increasingly requires the application of multidisciplinary teams and a unified concept of medicine across human and animal species lines.

9.4.3 Susceptible Population

Susceptibility of people to a given infection is a very important factor in infection spreading. Susceptibility to a disease is a biological property of tissues of a human or an animal, characterized by optimum conditions for the multiplication of pathogenic microorganisms. Susceptibility of an individual is affected by genetic factors, general resistance factors, and specific acquired immunity.

①Genetic factors in susceptibility to infectious diseases is not yet well understood. Genes do seem to play a role in the progression of HIV disease, and perhaps in individuals' susceptibility to meningococcal meningitis.

②General resistance factors include many body functions that we take for granted. Intact skin and mucous membranes help us resist disease, so does the gastric acid in our stomachs, the cilia in our respiratory tracts, and the cough reflex.

③Specific acquired immunity is the greatest influence on host susceptibility. This immunity is specific to a particular disease agent, and it may be acquired naturally or artificially.

• Natural immunity may be acquired by experiencing an infection, which is called "active natural immunity". Many diseases confer immunity after a single infection, but many others do not. A single bout of measles or chickenpox, for example, confers lifelong immunity to that disease. Influenza and salmonella are examples of infections that do not confer immunity and therefore may recur. Another mechanism of natural immunity is the transfer of antibodies from the mother to the newborn child via the placenta and/or breast milk. This is called "passive natural immunity", and it diminishes after varying lengths of time. It is very important in giving infants a good head start in life.

• Artificial immunity may be acquired using vaccines, toxoids and immune globulins. Artificially acquired immunity may also be active or passive. Artificially acquired active immunity may be produced by receiving a vaccine or toxoid to stimulate the immunity in an "active" manner, since the recipient responds by producing his/her antibodies. Artificially acquired passive immunity may be produced by receiving an antitoxin or immune globulin to confer "passive" immunity, essentially by borrowing the antibodies of other people. Passive immunity lasts for only a short time, while active immunity usually lasts much longer, even for a lifetime.

Apart from individual immunity, there also exists community immunity or herd immunity. Herd immunity is non-susceptibility of a community to a given infection. This type of immunity is created by specific prophylactic and other measures that are taken by health-care services, and also by the improvement of the well-being of the population. Susceptibility to disease, course of infection, and duration of immunity depend on the diet, ambient temperature, the physiological condition of an individual, and pre-existing or attending diseases. The immunologic structure of the population is the ratio of the number of people susceptibility to a given infection to the number of those non-susceptible to the disease. This ratio is determined by immunologic, serologic, and allergic reactions. If the number of susceptible people is not great, they are surrounded by many non-susceptible persons and the disease is thus not spread. For example, practical eradication of smallpox is due to compulsory vaccination of contacts around patients.

9.5　Prevention and Control of Communicable Diseases

The methods used to prevent communicable diseases in the past developed slowly through an empirical trial and error process. Today, the design of preventive strategies is based on a more deliberate process that relies on a detailed understanding of the pathogenesis of infection. For infection and disease to occur in a population, a process involving three related components must occur ①exposure to an infective agent; ②establishment of clinical disease in susceptible hosts; ③secondary dissemination of the infective agent through multiple routes. The process has been referred to as the "chain of infection". Therefore, prevention of communicable diseases can be carried out to break one or more of these links.

9.5.1　Strategies for Prevention of Communicable Diseases

①Prevention first, and the three-level prevention strategies should be adopted to comprehensively prevent and control infectious diseases.

②Strengthen the monitoring and management of infectious diseases. The contents of infectious disease surveillance include the incidence and death of infectious diseases, the types and characteristics of pathogens, the types and distribution of vector insects and animal hosts, the carrying status of pathogens, the level of population immunity and population data. If necessary, we should also conduct investigation on epidemic factors and epidemic law, and evaluate the effect of preventive measures. To formulate strict standards and management norms, supervise and manage pathogenic biological laboratories, infectious disease strains and virus seed banks, intensify the management of blood and blood products, biological products, biological specimens related to pathogenic organisms, and strengthen the training of personnel engaged in infectious diseases.

③Global Control of Infectious Diseases. Historically, plague, cholera, smallpox and influenza have occurred many times in the world. Therefore, the formulation of global control strategies for infectious diseases is not only necessary but also has achieved good results. In 1967, the WHO implemented the enhanced smallpox immunization program globally, and in 1980, smallpox was eliminated globally. In 1988 and 2001, the WHO launched the Global Polio Eradication Initiative and the Global Partnership to end tuberculosis, which also achieved remarkable results. Also, global control strategies for AIDS, malaria, leprosy, and tuberculosis have been launched to varying degrees around the world. During the SARS epidemic in 2003, the close cooperation of the whole world played a vital role in the victory of fighting against SARS.

9.5.2　Measures to Control Communicable Diseases

Besides antimicrobial agents, clean drinking water, reliable sewage disposal and vector control have contributed to the success of controlling many infectious diseases. The widespread application of vaccination programs has contributed further to the declining incidence of specific infections in most developed countries.

9.5.2.1   Safe Drinking Water

Safe and clean drinking water is an essential element of health security and underpins sustainable socio-economic development. Sewage is usually disposed of natural water bodies such as rivers and the sea. Separation of sewage and drinking water is probably the most effective means of preventing enteric infection. Drinking water is usually purified and rendered suitable for human consumption by a combination of filtration and chlorination. There are statutory regulations for drinking water standards in many countries. The provision of a safe potable water supply is a major priority for the world's population.

9.5.2.2   Safe Food Chain

The population may be at increased risk of infection if the food supply becomes contaminated. Food contamination can occur at any stage from the farm to the table. Preventing animal infections at the farm level can reduce food-borne illnesses. For example, reducing the amount of Salmonella in farm chickens by 50% (through better farm management) results in 50% lesser people getting sick from the bacteria. Salmonella-free chicken herds are becoming more common in some countries. Everyone on the food delivery chain must employ measures to keep food safe: farmer, processor, vendor and consumer. Safety at home is just as vital to prevent disease outbreaks. Women are primary targets for food safety education as they are responsible for house meals in many societies. The five keys to safer food are: to keep clean and wash hands before handling food, to separate raw and cooked food, to cool all foods thoroughly, to keep food at safe temperatures, and to use safe water and raw materials.

There are many methods to preserve food safely, including cold storage, canning, bottling and the use of preservative agents such as salt or sugar. The shift away from consumption of recently prepared fresh foodstuffs to packaged, convenience foods transported from distant places, with few preservatives, presents a range of opportunities for food-borne pathogens. Increased reliance on rapidly prepared foods from "fast food" outlets may also place the consumer at risk of food-borne infection because cooking times are often inadequate to successfully destroy gastrointestinal pathogens.

9.5.2.3   Action Against Vectors of Diseases

Many diseases are transmitted by either living or inanimate vectors. Inanimate objects can be cleaned, whereas living vectors present a different kind of target for preventive intervention. Insects play a particularly important role in the transmission of infectious diseases in warmer climates. Eradicating an insect vector or preventing contact with the human subject can be effective ways of preventing infection (e. g. , mosquito netting can be used to prevent malaria).

Poorly designed irrigation and water systems, inadequate housing, poor waste disposal and water storage, deforestation and loss of biodiversity, all may be contributing factors to most common vector-borne diseases including malaria, dengue and leishmaniasis. Rather than relying on a single method of vector control, IVM stresses the importance of first understanding the local vector ecology and local patterns of disease transmission, and subsequently of choosing the appropriate vector control tools from the following measures:

• Environmental management can reduce or eliminate vector breeding grounds through improved design or operation of water resources development projects.

• Biological controls (e. g. , bacterial larvicides and larvivorous fish) target and kill vector larvae without generating the ecological impacts of chemical use.

• Judicious use of chemical method when other measures are ineffective or not cost-effective, such as indoor residual sprays, space spraying, and use of chemical larvicides and adulticides. These may reduce disease transmission by shortening or interrupting the lifespan of vectors.

9.5.2.4   Private Hygiene

Although public and community health involves the supervision and surveillance of disease prevention strategies in the community, it is ultimately the responsibility of members of that community to make a strategy work. Effective prevention requires the education of every individual in basic preventive methods, e. g. , personal lavatory hygiene, food preparations and storage techniques, and prudent sexual behavior.

9.5.2.5   Vaccination

Considering the effectiveness of vaccination, WHO launched the Expanded Programme on Immunization (EPI) in 1974. The purpose of this program is to decrease morbidity and mortality caused by vaccine-preventable diseases in children since infections are major causes of death in children under 5 years old. Today, immunization saves more than 2.5 million lives of children per year. Due to increased immunization, polio has now been eradicated in most countries, and worldwide incidence was reduced from an estimated 350,000 cases in 1988 to just 223 cases in 2012. As of 2007, overall global measles deaths have fallen by 68%.

Vaccines include such types as:

①Live-attenuated vaccine prepared from attenuated non-pathogenic microorganisms.

②Inactivated vaccine prepared from inactive cultures of pathogenic microorganisms.

③Toxoids prepared by treating toxins (the poisons produced by microorganisms causing infectious diseases) with formaldehyde.

④Subunit vaccine isolated from microorganisms by various chemical methods.

⑤The conjugate vaccine created by covalently attaching a poor (polysaccharide organism) antigen to a carrier protein (preferably from the same microorganism).

⑥DNA vaccine genetically engineered by molecular techniques.

The Sabin polio vaccine consists of attenuated polio virus to provoke a protective immune reaction. This is achieved by intentionally exposing the subject to a modified strain of the viruses. Other examples are measles and BCG (bacilli Calmette-Guérin) vaccine.

With the development of molecular biology technology, further light has been thrown on the specific microbial components that are responsible for diseases. For example, modern hepatitis B vaccine contains HBsAg from yeast or mammalian cell cultures using recombinant DNA technology and have no risk of transmitting hepatitis B virus. A combination of hepatitis B immunoglobulin and an accelerated course of HBV vaccine prevent perinatal HBV transmission in around 90% of cases.

Ideally, immunization should take place before exposure to the infective agent to allow the development of protective immunity. However, some exposures inevitably take place in the absence of effective acquired immunity. Purified antibodies can offer protection to individuals at high risk of exposure. As recommended by WHO, postexposure prophylaxis with rabies immunoglobulin is required in case of severe exposure. Immunization of purified Vero cell vaccine (PVRV), purified primary chick embryo cell vaccine (PCECV), and human diploid cell vaccine (HDCV) are also needed as soon as possible.

Vaccination should be performed by physician or secondary medical personnel after a thorough examination to avoid possible contraindications or allergic reactions. The main contraindications to prophylactic vaccination are as follows:

①Acute fever, concurrent diseases attended by fever.

②Recently sustained infections.

③Chronic diseases such as tuberculosis, heart diseases, severe diseases of the kidneys, liver, stomach or other internal organs.

④The second half of pregnancy.

⑤First nursing period.

⑥Allergic diseases and states (bronchial asthma, hypersensitivity to some foods, and the like).

Vaccination can induce various reactions. These can be malaise, fever, nausea, vomiting, headache, and other general symptoms. A local reaction can also develop, e. g. , inflammation at the site of injection (hyperemia, odema, infiltration, regional lymphadenitis). Pathology can develop in response to vaccination. Such pathologies are regarded as postvaccination complications. They are divided into the following groups:

①Complications developing secondary to vaccination.

②Complications due to aseptic conditions of vaccination.

③Exacerbation of a pre-existing disease.

To prevent postvaccination complications, measures can be taken including strict observation of aseptic vaccination conditions, adherence to the schedule of vaccination, timely treatment of pathological states (anemia, rickets, skin diseases, etc.), timely revealing of contraindications to vaccination, and screening out the sick persons. All cases with severe reactions to vaccination should be reported to higher authorities.

9.5.2.6   Measures for the Reservoir of Infection

①For patients: early detection; early diagnosis; early report; early isolation; early treatment.

②For carriers: screening; physical examination; record.

③For susceptible contactors: quarantine.

④For animal reservoirs: sacrifice; vaccination; isolation.

All cases of infectious diseases or suspected cases should be recorded and reported to higher epidemiologic authorities within a certain time. The infectious patients must be isolated in proper time. Patients with plague, cholera, viral hepatitis, typhoid and paratyphoid fever, diphtheria, and similar contagious diseases should be immediately hospitalized. Patients should be handled in special ambulance cars that should be disinfected after the transportation of each patient. The patient delivered to the hospital must be given appropriate sanitary treatment before placing in the appropriate ward or an isolated room, if the diagnosis is not clear, or infection is mixed by its character. Special measures should be taken to prevent the spread of infection within the hospital. Persons cured of infectious diseases should be discharged from hospital after the alleviation of all clinical symptoms, and examination for the carrier state, specific for each infection. Persons who recovered from typhoid fever, paratyphoid, salmonellosis, dysentery should be observed in outpatient conditions. The term of observation depends on each particular disease.

Carriers of infection should be identified for medical examination and treatment. If the epidemiologic situation requires, the following groups of people should be examined for the carrier state:

①Persons contacting patients with typhoid fever, dysentery, paratyphoid, diphtheria, and meningococcal infection.

②Persons with a history of sustained typhoid fever, paratyphoid, and dysentery.

③Persons suspected of being a source of infection in the focus of infection.

The carriers must be immediately withdrawn from their occupation at food catering or children's institutions till they are completely cured and given multiple tests for the absence of the carrier state. Chronic carriers should be moved to other jobs that are not connected with food or children. Infection carriers must be regularly treated and observed according to special instructions.

If animals are the source of infection, measures are different. Veterinary measures should be taken concerning domestic animals. Animals with brucellosis should be slaughtered. Horses with glanders should also be killed. Food and materials obtained from diseased animals must be appropriately treated. Infected farms should be disinfected. Wild animals that are not the object of quarry must be destroyed, and measure for their isolation from man should be taken.

9.5.2.7　Measures to Stop Transmission

①Disinfection: prophylactic disinfection; disinfection of epidemic focus (concurrent)/ terminal.

②Disinsection and pest control.

The pathways by which infection can be transmitted are disrupted by acting on the transmission factors. Since intestinal infections are transmitted by the fecal-oral route, all preventive measures are aimed to preclude contact of the infected material with water, food, or hands. General sanitary measures should be taken constantly and universally, regardless of the presence or absence of infection in a given locality. Community hygiene is very important in the prevention of infection spread. The layout of settlements, housing conditions, the presence or absence of water supply and sewage systems are important factors in this respect. There are some important preventive measures, including permanent control of the water supply system, a correct selection of water body and the site of water intake, protection of the water intake zone, purification and decontamination of water. Soil protection from contamination with domestic wasters and sewage and timely cleaning of settlements are decisive measures against flies. Respiratory infections are easily transmitted from the source of infection to a susceptible population. The main measures are preventing overcrowding, adequate insolation and ventilation of enclosures, and the use of ultraviolet radiation for disinfection of air at medical and children's institutions.

9.5.2.8　Measures to Protect the Susceptible Population

①Immunization.

②Pharmaceutical prevention.

③Protective equipment.

General non-susceptibility of the population can be improved by better living and labor conditions, nutrition, physical training, health invigorating measures and by creating specific immunity through preventive vaccination.

9.5.3　Outbreaks and Epidemics

The occurrence of an epidemic implies that the existing preventive measures are inadequate and is often taken to indicate a need for further action. In general, the following approaches should be taken:

①Accurate diagnosis.

②Identification of the microbial cause.

③Confirmation of an epidemic, with preliminary surveillance data. This involves collecting information on the time of onset, personal details of each case and the geographical location.

④Production of a working hypothesis as to the likely cause, source and means of transmission.

⑤The intervention aimed to remove the source and interrupt transmission.

⑥Surveillance, to measure the effectiveness of actions taken and to indicate any need to modify those actions.

The efficiency of anti-epidemic measures taken in the focus of infection depends largely on the time when the source of infection (patient) is revealed and isolated from the surrounding people. Regardless of the character of the focus (family or community), measures should be taken toward the patient and persons who are in contact with the diseased subjects. As the diseased person is revealed, the following measures should be taken: disease diagnosis, case report, patient hospitalization or isolation in outpatient conditions, and specific therapy.

The focus should be examined by an epidemiologist or a rural physician. The purpose of the epidemiologic examination is to reveal the source and ways of infection transmission, to establish the boundaries of the focus, to determine the scope of disinfection and reveal contacts. A plan of immediate measures aimed to control and eradicate the focus should be made out.

Family members and contacts can help reveal the source of infection. Questioning usually begins by asking the patient's contact history. If a zoonotic focus is examined, possible contacts with the infected people or animals must be established. Information about previous travels to another city or village and visits of relatives or acquaintances from other districts should be revealed. It is very important to establish occupation of the diseases, conditions of his labor, living and nutrition conditions.

Material for microbiologic studies should be taken from the patient, the contacts, and, if necessary, animals and the surrounding objects (water, food, washings from equipment, various materials of animal origin, etc.).

The room where the patient is kept before hospitalization should be disinfected. After taking the patient to the hospital, or after his or her recovery from the disease (if the patient remained at home), the focus should be disinfected again. If the disease is transmitted by living vectors, disinfection must be carried out. Rodents must be exterminated in the focus of plague.

To stop the spread of infection and eradicate the focus of infection, specific preventive measures must be taken. Depending on indications the entire population in a given region or only separate persons who had contacts with the diseased must be vaccinated.

(Xiao Yanjie, Qu Quanying, Wang Hui, Zhao Jinshun)

Exercise

Chapter 10　Noncommunicable Disease Epidemiology

　　Noncommunicable diseases (NCDs) are currently the leading cause of death and disability worldwide. Once considered to be a health problem only for high-income countries, NCDs now account for more deaths than HIV, malaria, tuberculosis, diarrhea, and all other communicable diseases combined. NCDs have become one of the world's major public health problems, and understanding the epidemiology of NCDs is of great significance for the effective prevention and control of chronic diseases.

10.1　Introduction

10.1.1　Definition of Noncommunicable Diseases

　　NCDs are the major cause of adult mortality and morbidity worldwide. Also known as chronic diseases, NCDs are not passed from person to person and most do not include direct host-to-host transmission. The World Health Organization (WHO) identified NCDs as "Group II Diseases", a category that aggregates (based on the ICD-10 code) the following conditions/causes of death: malignant neoplasms, other neoplasms, diabetes mellitus, endocrine disorders, neuropsychiatric conditions, sense organ diseases, cardiovascular diseases, respiratory diseases (e. g. , chronic obstructive pulmonary disease [COPD], asthma, etc.), digestive diseases, genitourinary diseases, skin diseases, musculoskeletal diseases (e. g. , rheumatoid arthritis), congenital anomalies (e. g. , cleft palate, Down's syndrome), and oral conditions (e. g. , dental caries).

　　WHO identified four main diseases to be dominant in NCD mortality and morbidity: cardiovascular diseases (including heart disease and stroke), diabetes, cancer, and chronic respiratory diseases (including COPD and asthma).

10.1.2　The Health and Socioeconomic Impacts of NCDs

10.1.2.1　The Health Impacts

　　Health systems are facing an increasing burden associated with NCDs. Globally, WHO estimates NCDs contribute to 82 percent of premature deaths in low and middle-income countries. In 2017, NCDs caused 73.4 percent of all deaths (41.1 million) in the world. About half of them affected the population under age 70. Five major NCDs (diabetes, cardiovascular diseases, cancer, chronic respiratory diseases, and mental disorders) account for 86 percent of deaths.

10. 1. 2. 2   The Socioeconomic Impacts

Concerns about the economic impact of NCDs are growing due to the high prevalence and chronic course of these diseases over the lifespan of the population. NCDs deprive individuals of their health and productive potential. The burden of chronic diseases may invariably challenge an individual or household income and savings and compete with investment activities. Chronic diseases reduce life expectancy and ultimately economic productivity, thus depleting the quality and quantity of a country's labor force. This may result in lower national output in national income (gross domestic product [GDP] and gross national income). An extreme simplification of these channels and linkages is presented in Figure 10. 1.

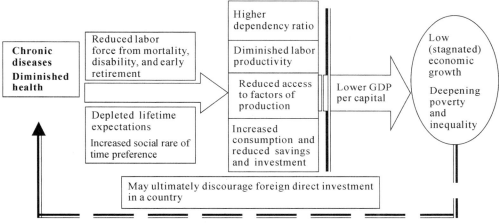

Figure 10. 1   The Socioeconomic Impacts of NCDs

10. 1. 3   Characteristics of NCDs

NCDs are characterized by uncertain etiology, multiple factors, a long latency period, a prolonged course of illness, non-contagious origin, functional disability, and Occasional incurability.

Unlike communicable diseases, most NCDs do not have a single and exact cause of disease. Their etiology is manifold and complex with a long latency period. NCDs generally last a long time and progress slowly, and thus they are sometimes also referred to as chronic diseases. They can arise from environmental exposures or from genetically determined abnormalities, which may be evident at birth or which may become apparent later in life.

NCDs that arise from inherited genetic abnormalities often leave an individual ill-equipped to survive without treatment. Examples of the inherited disease include cystic fibrosis, Down syndrome, and inborn errors of metabolism, which are present at birth. Inherited diseases that emerge in adulthood include Huntington disease and certain forms of cancer (e. g. , familial breast cancer involving inherited mutations in the BRCA1 or BRCA2 genes).

10. 1. 4   Risk Factors of NCDs

Factors including age, gender, genetics, exposure to air pollution, smoking, unhealthy diet, and physical inactivity can lead to hypertension and obesity, further increasing the risk of many other NCDs. WHO's World Health Report 2002 identified five important risk factors for NCDs in the top ten risks to health, namely elevated blood pressure, elevated cholesterol, tobacco use, alcohol consumption, and being overweight. Other factors associated with NCDs include a person's economic and social conditions, also known as the social determinants of health.

It has been estimated that if the primary risk factors were eliminated, 80 percent of heart disease, stroke, and type 2 diabetes and 40 percent of cancer cases could be prevented. Interventions targeting the main risk factors could have a significant impact on reducing the burden of disease worldwide. Efforts focusing on a better diet and increased physical activity have been shown to reduce the risk of NCDs.

NCDs affect people of all age groups, regions, and countries. Of the "premature" deaths due to NCDs, over 85 percent are estimated to occur in low-and middle-income countries. Children, adults, and the elderly are all vulnerable to the risk factors, namely unhealthy diets, physical inactivity, exposure to tobacco smoke, and harmful use of alcohol.

These diseases are driven by forces that include rapid unplanned urbanization, globalization of unhealthy lifestyles, and population aging. Unhealthy diets and physical inactivity may present as metabolic risk factors that can lead to cardiovascular diseases: high blood pressure, increased blood glucose, elevated blood lipids, and obesity.

10. 2   Epidemiological Characteristics of NCDs

10. 2. 1   Global Epidemiological Characteristics

The Global Burden of Disease (GBD) Study reported that NCDs were collectively responsible for 73. 4 percent of total deaths worldwide in 2017. NCDs account for 53 percent of global years of life lost. The largest numbers of deaths from NCDs were estimated for cardiovascular diseases (17. 8 million deaths), cancer (9. 56 million deaths), and chronic respiratory diseases (3. 91 million deaths). From 2007 to 2017, the total numbers of cancer deaths increased by 25. 4, cardiovascular disease deaths increased by 21. 1 percent, chronic respiratory diseases increased by 15. 8 percent, and diabetes mellitus deaths increased by 34. 7 percent.

10. 2. 2   Epidemiological Characteristics in China

According to GBD 2015, the mortality rate of chronic diseases among Chinese residents was 594. 3/100,000, accounting for 87. 2 percent of all deaths. In 2015, the deaths caused by four major chronic diseases (cardiovascular and cerebrovascular disease, malignant tumor, COPD, and diabetes) accounted for 88.5 percent of the total deaths from chronic diseases and 77.1 percent of total deaths.

The GBD results showed that disability-adjusted life year (DALY) caused by chronic diseases was 2.8 million years in China in 2015, accounting for 81.3 percent of the total DALY in China, and 19.1 percent of the global DALY, representing an increase of 16.7 percent compared with 1990 (Figure 10.2).

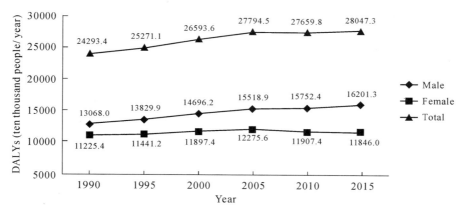

Figure 10.2   The Trend of DALY Caused by Chronic Diseases in China from 1990 to 2015

10.2.3   Epidemiological Characteristics of NCD Risk Factors

Four major modifiable factors are the main drivers in the rise of NCDs: tobacco use, the harmful use of alcohol, unhealthy diets, and physical inactivity.

10.2.3.1   Tobacco Use

Smoking contains more than 7,000 chemical constituents, of which hundreds are harmful substances and at least 69 are carcinogens. Smoking is an important risk factor for the occurrence of and death from malignant tumors, chronic respiratory diseases, coronary heart disease, stroke, aortic aneurysm, and peripheral vascular diseases.

Smokers have an 18-fold higher risk of developing lung cancer than non-smokers. Smoking is associated with 90 percent of male lung cancer deaths and 80 percent of female lung cancer deaths. In addition to lung cancer, ample evidence suggests that smoking can also cause oral, laryngeal, esophageal, gastric, liver, pancreatic, colorectal, renal, bladder, and cervical cancer.

Smoking is a major risk factor for COPD and bronchial asthma, especially in females. 90 percent of the deaths of females with COPD can be attributed to smoking. Ample evidence suggests that smoking can lead to asthma or asthma-like symptoms in adolescents and increase their risk of respiratory infections and tuberculosis.

Smoking is also an independent risk factor for cardiovascular and cerebrovascular diseases. Among the nine independent risk factors leading to coronary heart disease, smoking ranked second; high cholesterol ranked first.

Second-hand smoke exposure can lead to lung cancer, cardiovascular and cerebrovascular diseases, and other serious diseases in non-smokers. Second-hand smoke exposure is particularly harmful to the health of pregnant women, infants, and children and increases the risk of sudden neonatal death syndrome, otitis media, and low birth weight.

The global Adult Tobacco Survey in 2015 shows that the current smoking rate is 27.7 percent in Chinese residents aged 15 and over. Among them, the smoking rate in males is as high as 52.1 percent; the smoking rate in females is maintained at a low level of 2.7 percent. No statistical difference is present in the current smoking rate between urban and rural population. More than one million people in China die from tobacco-related diseases every year, accounting for 12 percent of all deaths.

10.2.3.2　Alcohol Use

According to WHO, dangerous drinking refers to the drinking behavior of male drinkers whose daily intake of pure alcohol is greater than or equal to 41g and less than 61g, and female drinkers whose daily intake of pure alcohol is greater than or equal to 21g and less than 41g. Harmful drinking refers to the drinking behavior of male drinkers whose daily intake of pure alcohol is equal to 61g or more, and female drinkers whose daily intake of pure alcohol is equal to 41g or more.

Excessive drinking is closely related to chronic diseases. Long-term excessive drinking is an important risk factor for cardiovascular and cerebrovascular diseases. Epidemiological studies confirmed that 5—7 percent of hypertension was attributed to heavy drinking. Alcohol consumption and blood pressure show a dose-effect relationship. Drinking also increases the risk of stroke, and it is closely related to dyslipidemia and the risk of diabetes.

10.2.3.3　Unhealthy Diet

An unhealthy diet includes high fat, high sugar, high salt, inadequate intake of fresh vegetables and fruits, eating quickly, high-temperature food, overeating habits, etc. WHO points out that an unhealthy diet is one of the main risk factors for chronic diseases. An unhealthy diet is closely related to chronic diseases such as cardiovascular and cerebrovascular diseases, diabetes mellitus, malignant tumors, and obesity.

A high-fat diet is an important risk factor for chronic diseases in Chinese adults. A change in the proportion of fat in the diet has little effect on the glucose fluctuation in normal-weight individuals but has a great influence on the glucose fluctuation in overweight and obese individuals. In overweight and obese individuals on a high-fat diet for three days, 50 percent of dietary fat content could significantly affect the fluctuation of glucose compared with 30 percent of dietary fat content for three days. The total fat intake in the diet, especially the intake of saturated fatty acids, has been positively correlated with the incidence of atherosclerosis. Along with an increase in the fat energy supply ratio, the fasting blood sugar, total cholesterol, and triglyceride levels significantly increase. In the elderly, a high-fat diet affected the microcirculation, causing atherosclerosis and hyperlipidemia. Saturated fatty acid intake is positively correlated with the occurrence of colorectal cancer. Excessive saturated fatty acid intake cannot be fully absorbed by the small intestine. Residual fatty acid enters the colon. Fatty acid and secondary cholic acid (mainly lithocholic acid) in the intestinal cavity interfere with the integrity of intestinal epithelium, leading to epithelial tissue damage and cell proliferation, thus inducing the occurrence of tumors.

A high-sugar diet can cause hyperinsulinemia, insulin resistance, hypertension, and tachycardia. When the ratio of carbohydrate intake to total energy is more than 60 percent, the prevalence of hypertension increases significantly. Studies have shown that a high-sugar diet not only increases waist circumference, but also may increase the risk of breast cancer. Excessive carbohydrate intake can rapidly increase the body's glycemic production index and blood sugar load, which can lead to cell division, increase the level of blood estrogen, and promote the occurrence of breast cancer.

A high-salt diet is harmful to health. It is an important reason for high blood pressure and the prevalence of hypertension. It is also an important risk factor for chronic diseases such as coronary heart disease and stroke. In the long term, a high-salt diet may induce gastric cancer, asthma, and osteoporosis caused by increased urinary calcium excretion.

10. 2. 3. 4   Physical Inactivity

With increasing urbanization, the popularization of the Internet and smart devices, physical activity has declined, particularly in occupational settings, and sedentary behavior has increased. Inadequate physical activity is an independent risk factor for cardiovascular and cerebrovascular diseases (especially coronary disease), type 2 diabetes, obesity, and other chronic diseases. The risk of diabetes mellitus and cerebrovascular disease increase by 73 percent and 80 percent in those who sit still for more than 4 hours a day and watch TV for more than 3 hours a day. A long-term sedentary lifestyle and lack of exercise could impair human physiology and lead to decreased immune function, thereby increasing the risk of cardiovascular disease, digestive disease, bone and joint disease, metabolic disease, and colorectal cancer, breast cancer, osteoporosis, depression and anxiety disorders, and more.

10. 3   Prevention and Control of NCDs

10. 3. 1   Prevention Strategy

NCD prevention is accomplished by choosing strategies and measures that have been proven to be effective with scientific evidence regarding disease etiology, physiological functions, and the natural history of the disease. Prevention aims to avoid the occurrence, development, or deterioration of disease and to improve the quality of life.

NCDs have multiple causes, including genetic, environmental and psychosocial factors. These factors depend on and interact with each other. NCDs cannot be prevented by biomedical methods alone; psychosocial factors must also be included.

The following strategies and measures should be considered for preventing and controlling NCDs:

①Applying prevention strategies, combined with comprehensive measures including treatment.

②Changing and avoiding unhealthy lifestyle choices and behaviors, such as smoking, drinking, unhealthy diets, mental stress, physical inactivity, and so on.

③Applying community-based health education strategies.

④Beginning prevention during childhood and emphasizing continuous health management throughout life.

⑤Implementing primary prevention, followed by secondary prevention and tertiary prevention.

⑥Using both the whole population strategy and high-risk population strategy as appropriate.

10.3.1.1   WHO-Recommended Strategies for Preventing NCDs

Primary health care (PHC) can be defined as follows: essential health care based on practical, scientifically sound, and socially acceptable methods and technology, made universally accessible to individuals and families in the community. It is through their full participation and at a cost that the community and the country can afford to maintain at every stage of their development in the spirit of self-reliance and self-determination.

In other words, PHC is an approach to health beyond the traditional health care system that focuses on health equity-producing social policy. PHC includes all areas that play a role in health, such as access to health services, environment, and lifestyles.

The ultimate goal of primary health care is better health for all. WHO has identified five key elements to achieving that goal:

①Reducing exclusion and social disparities in health (universal coverage reforms).

②Organizing health services around people's needs and expectations (service delivery reforms).

③Integrating health into all sectors (public policy reforms).

④Pursuing collaborative models of policy dialogue (leadership reforms).

⑤Increasing stakeholder participation.

Behind these elements lie a series of basic principles identified in the Alma Ata Declaration that should be formulated in national policies to launch and sustain PHC as part of a comprehensive health system and in coordination with other sectors.

Equitable distribution of health care—according to this principle, primary care and other services to meet the main health problems in a community must be provided equally to all individuals regardless of their gender, age, color, urban/rural location, and social class/caste.

Community participation—due to its grassroots nature and emphasis on self-sufficiency, community participation is considered sustainable compared to targeted (or vertical) approaches, which depend on international development assistance. Community participation makes the most of local, national and other available resources.

Health workforce development—comprehensive health care relies on an adequate number and distribution of trained physicians, nurses, allied health professionals, community health workers, and others working as a health team and supported at the local and referral levels.

Use of appropriate technology—medical technology should be accessible, affordable, feasible, and culturally acceptable to the community. Examples of appropriate technology include refrigerators for vaccine cold storage. Less appropriateness could include, in many settings, body scanners or heart-lung machines, which benefit only a small minority concentrated in urban areas. These devices are generally not accessible to the poor but draw a large share of resources.

Multi-sectional approach—health cannot be improved by intervention within just the formal health sector; other sectors are equally important in promoting the health and self-reliance of communities. These sectors include, at minimum: agriculture (e. g. , food security); education; communication (e. g. , concerning prevailing health problems and the methods of preventing and controlling them); housing; public works (e. g. , ensuring an adequate supply of safe water and basic sanitation); rural development; industry; community organizations (including Panchayats or local governments, voluntary organizations, etc.).

In summary, PHC recognizes that health care is not a short-lived intervention, but an ongoing process of improving people's lives and alleviating the underlying socioeconomic conditions that contribute to poor health. The principles link health and development, advocating political interventions, rather than passive acceptance of economic conditions.

10. 3. 1. 2　Three Levels of Preventive Measures for Chronic Diseases

(1)Primary Prevention

Primary prevention, also called causal prevention, is a measure that targets the cause of disease. Primary prevention denotes an action taken to prevent the development of a disease in a person who is well and does not (yet) have the disease in question. Primary prevention is our ultimate goal. However, although we intend to prevent diseases from occurring in human populations, we lack the biologic, clinical, and epidemiologic data on which we could base effective primary prevention programs for many diseases. Primary prevention activities fall into two major categories: health promotion and health protection.

①Health promotion. Health promotion is achieved by creating a healthy environment that allows people to avoid or reduce exposure to pathogenic factors, changing the body's susceptibility to protect people from disease. Health promotion enables people to increase control over their health and its determinants, and thereby to improve their health. It includes health education, self-care, environmental protection, and surveillance.

②Health protection. Health protection includes measures for preventing a particular disease or health condition, or preventing disease in a specific high-risk population, through targeted preventive methods that eliminate the effects of the causes of disease.

③The whole population strategy and the high-risk population strategy. Two possible approaches to prevention are the whole population strategy and the high-risk population strategy. In the whole population strategy, a preventive measure is widely applied to an entire population. For example, prudent dietary advice for preventing coronary disease or advice against smoking may be provided to an entire population. An alternate approach is to target a high-risk population with a preventive measure. Thus, cholesterol screening in children might be restricted to children from high-risk families. A measure that will be applied to an entire population must be relatively inexpensive and noninvasive. A measure to be applied to a high-risk subgroup of the population may be more expensive, invasive, or complex. The whole population strategy can be considered a public health approach, whereas the high-risk population strategy more often requires a clinical action to identify the high-risk group to be targeted. In most situations, a combination of both approaches is ideal.

(2)Secondary Prevention

Secondary prevention, or so-called "triple early prevention", refers to the early detection, timely diagnosis, and prompt treatment of disease. It involves identifying people in whom a disease has already developed but who do not yet display clinical signs and symptoms of the illness. This period in the life cycle of a disease is called the preclinical phase of the illness. Once a person develops clinical signs or symptoms, it is generally assumed the person will seek medical care. With secondary prevention, the objective is to detect the disease earlier than it would have been detected with standard care. By detecting the disease at an early stage in its evolution, often through screening, it is hoped that treatment will be easier and/or more effective. For example, routine stool testing for occult blood can detect treatable colon cancer early in its natural history. The rationale for secondary prevention is that if we can identify disease earlier in its development than would ordinarily occur, intervention measures will be more effective. Perhaps we can prevent mortality or complications of the disease and use less invasive or less costly treatment to do so.

(3)Tertiary Prevention

Tertiary prevention, also called "clinical prevention", is employed to prevent complications in those who have already developed signs and symptoms of an illness and have been diagnosed. This is generally achieved through prompt and appropriate treatment of the illness combined with ancillary approaches, such as physical therapy, designed to prevent complications such as joint contractures.

10. 3. 2 Preventive Measures for NCDs

Two types of preventive measures may be applied for NCDs: preventive treatments and reducing the level of risk factors. Both measures rely heavily on epidemiologic knowledge. Benjamin Franklin once said, "An ounce of prevention is worth a pound of cure". —wise words that are applicable when speaking of preventive measures to keep chronic health issues at bay. The good news is that a growing body of research highlights how healthy lifestyles— good eating habits, regular exercise, and routine screenings—can be instrumental in preventing chronic illnesses. Tackling the risk factors will therefore not only save lives; it will also provide a huge boost for countries' economic development.

There are many preventive measures for chronic diseases. In preparation for the UN High-Level Meeting, WHO identified a set of evidence-based "best buy" interventions that are not only highly cost-effective but also feasible and appropriate to implement within the constraints of the local health systems of low- and middle-income countries (Table 10.1). Of course, many other interventions exist to reduce chronic disease at the population or individual level that, while not meeting all "best buy" criteria, may still contribute to a comprehensive public health response to the challenge of NCDs. WHO has developed a costing tool to enable countries to add or substitute interventions according to national needs or priorities.

Table 10.1   "Best Buy" Interventions

Risk Factor/Disease	Interventions
Tobacco use	①Tax increases ②Smoke-free indoor workplaces and public places ③Health information and warnings ④Bans on tobacco advertising, promotion, and sponsorship
Harmful alcohol use	①Tax increases ②Restricted access to retailed alcohol ③Bans on alcohol advertising
Unhealthy diet and physical inactivity	①Reduced salt intake in food ②Replacement of trans fat with polyunsaturated fat ③Public awareness through mass media on diet and physical activity
Cardiovascular disease (CVD) and diabetes	①Counseling and multi-drug therapy for people with a high risk of developing heart attacks and strokes (including those with established CVD) ②Treatment of heart attacks with aspirin
Cancer	①Hepatitis B immunization to prevent liver cancer (already scaled up) ②Screening and treatment of pre-cancerous lesions to prevent cervical cancer

10.3.3   NCD Management Model

In practice, the most effective strategies for disease control and prevention are based on the epidemic background and characteristics of the disease in a particular area, the specific situation and needs of this area, and on the human and organizational resources available.

The strategy may be global, national, or regional, and it may focus on multiple diseases and health problems in the whole population or on a single disease.

10.3.3.1 NCD Prevention Models

Since the late 19th century, the biomedical model has undoubtedly become the mainstream medical model. However, beginning in the 1960s, the biomedical model has been questioned by some scholars. Awareness is more prevalent that, although traditional medicine might promote disease treatment, it is not conducive to maintaining and promoting health. The biopsychosocial model regards health as a dynamic state of complete physical, mental, spiritual, and social well-being, and not merely the absence of disease or infirmity. It is also the outcome of the combined effect of factors related to individual, environment, and public health support services.

The main determinants of health include four broad elements (Figure 10.3):

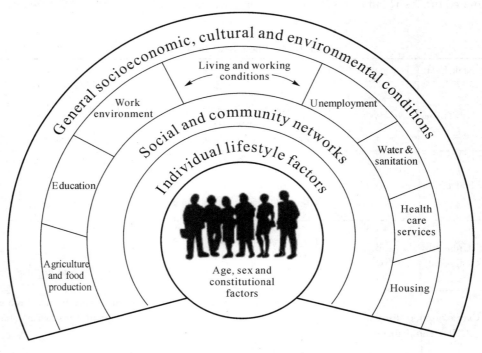

Figure 10.3   The Main Determinants of Health

①Human biology: biological, genetic, physiological, immunological, etc.

②Environment: natural environment, social environment, and psychological environment.

③Lifestyle: hobbies, sexual behavior, customs, psychological stress, etc.

④Health care organization.

10.3.3.2 The Improved NCD Management Model

(1) Integrated Evidence-Based NCD Management Model

This model describes four interacting system components, namely, health care providers, the health care system, community partners, and patients with their families. The main feature of this model is the integration of services provided by nurses, community health care workers, and traditional health practitioners. The model proposes a well-established clinical information system to allow health care providers access to more informed patient care. The health care system based on this model will be tasked to organize health care in rural areas to improve management and prevention of chronic illnesses. Support systems, including supervisory visits to clinics, provision of medical equipment, and the training of health care providers, should be provided. The model also emphasizes contributions from community partners, in the form of better leadership to mobilize and coordinate resources for chronic care. District and provincial health departments can support this productive interaction by reorganizing health services to give local officials a role in leadership and to improve community participation.

(2) Integrated Chronic Disease Management Model

The integrated chronic disease management (ICDM) model uses a public health approach to empower individuals to take responsibility for their health while simultaneously intervening at a community/population and health-service level. The ICDM aims to achieve optimal clinical outcomes for patients with chronic communicable and non-communicable diseases in an efficient and cost-effective manner, as an innovative response to the growing burden of disease.

The ICDM consists of four inter-related intervention phases (facility re-organization, clinical supportive management, assisted self-support, and strengthening of support systems and structures outside the facility) that interact at the health-service level, individual patient level and the community/population level to ensure a seamless transition to assisted self-management within the community. Strong stewardship and ownership at all levels of the health system is the most critical success factor for the four intervention phases.

10.3.3.3   NCD Management Model in China

At the founding of People's Republic of China, a three-tiered system of health and disease control was established, step by step, under the Ministry of Health of the central government. The system includes health and anti-epidemic stations in the provinces, regions, and counties, and in large-scale enterprises and mines; the committee for patriotic public health campaign; maternity and pediatric health care centers; centers for control of different specialized diseases such as occupational diseases, endemic diseases, tuberculosis, and leprosy, and institutes for health control such as food hygiene, environmental health, school hygiene, and so on in the provinces and cities. Entry-exit inspection and quarantine bureaus have also been instituted at the ports and airports.

The national health campaign is a mass movement under government leadership, in collaboration with various agencies, and with the participation of the Chinese population. Since its inception, it has proven to be a very effective model of public health. In the 1950s, the central mission of this movement was to eradicate four hazards (flies, mosquitoes, mice, and cockroaches). In the 1960s, the main tasks turned toward controlling water (waste and drinking water), improving the quality of drinking water, reconstructing toilets and livestock farms, redesigning cooking furnaces, and remediating the environment. In the late 1970s, the important objectives were to control environmental health in the cities, further emphasizing water control and reconstructing toilets in the countryside and health education for the entire population of China. By the end of 1997, the water supply system had benefited 850 million people, and 25.4 percent of excrement and urine was treated.

The Healthy China 2030 Plan, released by the Communist Party of China Central Committee and the State Council on October 25, 2016, aims to enhance its people's health through promoting healthy lifestyles, optimizing health services, improving health security, building a healthy environment, and developing health industries. The plan covers topics such as public health services, environmental management, medical industry, and food and drug safety based on the country's new development concepts: innovation, environmental concern, coordination, and open and shared growth.

(Zhou Zhiheng, Hu Fulan, He Fei, Wang Hui, Zhao Jinshun)

Exercise

Chapter 11   Molecular Epidemiology

Molecular epidemiology is a discipline that uses molecular microbiology tools to study the distribution and determinants of diseases in human populations, and has grown rapidly in the last decade. Our understanding of molecular epidemiology has evolved with technological advancements made in molecular biology. In this chapter, we define molecular epidemiology and introduce its main research content, research methods, applications and outlooks.

11.1   Introduction

11.1.1   Definition of Molecular Epidemiology

Molecular epidemiology is a new branch of epidemiology that combines traditional epidemiology with emerging biological technologies, especially with molecular biology techniques. It mainly clarifies the law of disease occurrence and development, and its influencing factors at the molecular level to solve a series of difficulties encountered in traditional epidemiology effectively. "Molecule" in molecular epidemiology refers to the application of molecular biology theory and technology to solve epidemiological problems, while "epidemiology" refers to the use of epidemiological research methods to explore molecular biotechnology from the perspective of epidemiology. The results detected by molecular biotechnology are translated into an interpretation of the etiology, pathogenesis and diagnosis of the disease in the population. Therefore, molecular epidemiology can be defined as the application of the techniques of molecular biology to the study of the epidemiology of the disease in human populations.

Molecular epidemiological studies aim to establish causality and biological plausibility for associations between exposure and disease. Before this, the determined biomarkers must be identified. Biomarkers are cellular, subcellular and substances of molecular levels that are measurable from the continuous process of exposure to disease, which can reflect functional or structural changes.

11.1.2   The Emergence and Development of Molecular Epidemiology

11.1.2.1   Background

Epidemiology has always played an important role in the prevention and treatment of diseases, the research and control of disease risk factors, and new problems in disease prevention. However, since the late period of 20th century, with the deepening of disease pre-

vention and control and health promotion and the increasing demand for health, epidemiological research and application have encountered new challenges.

First of all, there are some new problems in the prevention of infectious diseases, mainly manifested as follows: ①The wide application of antibiotics, results in the emergence of a
variety of drug-resistant pathogens, leading to difficulties for traditional epidemiological
methods to develop better preventive and control measures. ②The pathogens continue to
show diversity and variability, and the epidemiology and transmission mechanism of infectious diseases are becoming more and more complicated. ③The emergence of new infectious
diseases has forced us to use the fastest technical methods in the earliest stages to clarify the
causes of diseases and provide a basis for the prevention and control of infectious diseases.
For chronic non-communicable diseases, traditional epidemiological methods based on the
"black box principle" have been unable to meet the requirements for disease prevention and
health promotion in the new era. Also, basic medicine developed rapidly in the late 20th
century, especially in biochemistry and molecular biology. Many pathogenesis and causal
hypotheses were proposed from the molecular and gene levels. This requires exploring its a-
vailability as a biomarker to screen high-risk populations and evaluate their effects on disease
control.

Considering above problems, researchers began to realize that if an intermediate event
in the occurrence and development of diseases, not just the outcome, was used as a measurement index to study the distribution characteristics, influencing factors and intervention
effects of the disease, it will greatly improve the effectiveness of epidemiological research.
How to measure intermediate events? The development of molecular biology, especially the
emergence of molecular biology techniques, has brought about the possibility of solving
these problems. In the late 20th century, with the deepening of research on gene and protein
levels, molecular biology theory and technology have developed rapidly. The level of detection and identification of molecules has been greatly improved.

The rapid development of these theories and techniques has given new features to epidemiology. Researchers have begun to use biomarkers as evaluation indicators to solve intermediate events and susceptibility measurement problems in the process of disease development. The influencing factors and the best prevention strategies eventually formed a new
discipline, namely molecular epidemiology.

11. 1. 2. 2   Development Process

In 1972, Kilbourne et al. presented a report entitled "Molecular Epidemiology of Influenza" at the 10th Annual Meeting of the American Society of Infectious Diseases. For the
first time, the term "molecular epidemiology" was used. The related paper was published in
Journal of Infectious Diseases in 1973. In 1977, French scholar Higginson made a preliminary explanation for molecular epidemiology, using sophisticated techniques for epidemiological studies of biological materials. In 1982, Perera and Weinstein proposed "cancer molecular epidemiology", which believed that cancer molecular epidemiology was a method that u-

ses advanced laboratory techniques combined with analytical epidemiology to study tumor causes at the biochemical or molecular level. With the development of the Human Genome Project, Khoury and Dorman first proposed the concept of human genome epidemiology in 1998.

In the early 1980s, China began to conduct molecular epidemiological studies, limited to infectious diseases, such as studies on rotavirus diarrhea, Escherichia coli diarrhea. In 1992, the Chinese Journal of *Epidemiology* systematically introduced the "Molecular Epidemiology Research and Application". Its main content was monographed in the chapter "Molecular Epidemiology" in *Modern Epidemiology Methods and Applications* edited by Zeng Guang in 1994. The National Conference on Molecular Epidemiology was held in 1998, 2004, 2012, 2015 and 2018, respectively. Molecular epidemiology has since become one of the most active areas of epidemiological research in China.

After more than 30 years of development, molecular epidemiology has formed a relatively complete theory and method system, playing an increasingly important role in disease prevention and control. The development of molecular epidemiology in the past decade has been mainly characterized by richer research content, diverse methods and expanding application scope.

11.1.3　Relationship with Traditional Epidemiology

The relationship between traditional epidemiology and molecular epidemiology can be seen in Figure 11.1. Traditional epidemiology mainly uses case-control studies or cohort studies to assess whether there is a association between exposure and disease. Molecular epidemiology is the process of conducting related research by detecting biomarkers.

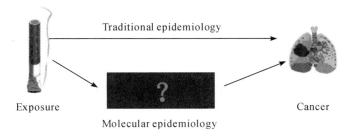

Figure 11.1　Relationship Between Traditional Epidemiology and Molecular Epidemiology

Although molecular epidemiology has developed rapidly in recent years, there are still many immature areas due to its terminology, and it needs constant improvement and development. At the same time, the definition of many disciplines is correspondingly revised as it develops. We believe that the definition of molecular epidemiology will become more perfect and correct as its theory continues to enrich and practice.

11. 2　The Research Content

11. 2. 1　The Study of Biomarkers

The term "biomarker" is a portmanteau of "biological marker". In 1998, the National Institutes of Health Biomarkers Definitions Working Group defined a biomarker as "a characteristic that is objectively measured and evaluated as an indicator of normal biological processes, pathogenic processes, or pharmacologic responses to a therapeutic intervention". Of late, the International Programme on Chemical Safety, has defined a biomarker as "any substance, structure, or process that can be measured in the body or its products and influence or predict the incidence of outcome or disease" in 2015. In practice, biomarkers include tools and technologies that can aid in understanding the prediction, cause, diagnosis, progression, regression, or outcome of treatment of the disease.

The application of biomarkers in the diagnosis and management of cardiovascular diseases, infections, immunological and genetic disorders, and cancer is well known. In the area of cardiovascular diseases, the research involved with molecular epidemiology has been conducted for decades. For example, in the 1960s, elevated serum cholesterol level (a biomarker of biologically effective dose) was linked to the risk of ischemic heart disease.

Biomarkers are generally classified into three major groups: biomarkers of exposure, effect, and susceptibility. Although exposure biomarkers are often described as a separate topic from effect biomarkers, there is only a semantic distinction between these two biomarkers. There are many overlapping continuums leading from exposure to a toxic agent (such as carcinogens), metabolism (activation or deactivation), adduction to proteins or deoxyribonucleic acid (DNA) (i. e., formation of links by active metabolites), DNA alterations (such as mutations or chromosome damage), onset of disease, and finally, progression of disease (Figure 11. 2).

As listed in Table 11. 1, the utility of several molecular-based assays as a marker of both exposure and effect is discussed. For example, a DNA adduct in a range of cell types has been used for decades to monitor exposure to environmental carcinogens. From this perspective, it can be classified as an exposure biomarker. However, there is evidence pointing out that endogenous oxidant-induced DNA adduct may contribute significantly to aging and cancer. In this respect, DNA adduct can be regarded as an effect biomarker. Therefore, DNA adduct is not comfortably forced exclusively into one or another category. Nevertheless, the categorization, if held lightly, can be helpful in descriptive purposes as well as informing discussions of disease mechanisms. The section will present generally accepted definitions of the three categories of biomarkers, and examples of the various categories of biomarkers are given.

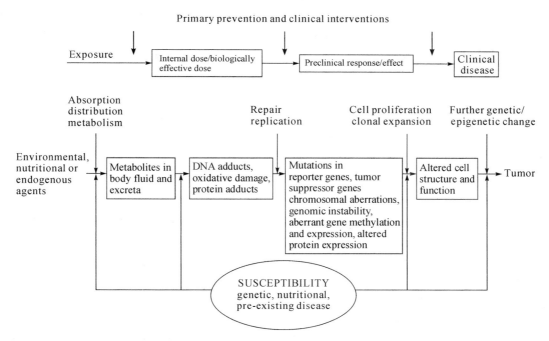

Figure 11. 2   The Relationship Between Exposure, Exposure Biomarkers, Effect Biomarkers,
Medical Surveillance, and the Onset of Disease

Table 11. 1   **Examples of Biomarkers of Exposure and Effect**[*]

Biomarker	Exposure Biomarker	Effect Biomarker
DNA adducts	As a result of exogenous exposure	Absorption, distribution, metabolism, and DNA repair
Epigenetic modifications	CpG-promoter sequence methylation, histone modification, and chromatin remodeling	Alterations in the balance of methylation are related to gene transcriptional silencing
Transcriptomics	Alterations in gene expression vary depending on the type of exposure	Changes in gene expression profiles in response to chronic exposure
Proteomics	Albumin and hemoglobin adducts; changes in protein structure because of exposure	Changes in protein expression because of exposure (i. e. , altered growth factors and cytokines)
Metabolomics	Accumulation of metabolites of exposure agents	Changes in the metabolic capacity because of exposure or disease

* Modified based on *Handbook of Epidemiology*

11. 2. 2   Exposure Biomarkers

External exposure is the measured concentration of the chemicals in an individual's immediate environment. While questionnaires offer a historical account of the exposure, direct measurement of the alleged chemical in various exposure media (air, water, soil, or food) can give accurate information regarding the "dose" of the exposure. However, a measurement of "internal" dose may provide a more objective measure of "true" exposure than "external" concentration. When the chemical is identified in tissues or body fluids, it becomes a biomarker for the internal dose, and is generally called an "exposure biomarker".

Exposure biomarkers are the actual chemicals, or chemical metabolites, or the product of interaction with target molecules that can be measured in the target organ or its surrogate to determine different characteristics of an organism's exposure. Exposure biomarkers can provide an improved metric of exposure compared with levels in ambient air, food, or water. For example, a history of lead exposure can be strengthened by measurement of lead in the environment, but the best indication of the dose of exposure may be determined in blood and tissues (hair, nails, teeth, etc.). The advantage of using biomarkers is that such use can overcome the problem of limited recall or lack of awareness of an exposure. Besides, biomarkers can correct errors resulting from variation in individual absorption or metabolism by focusing on a later step in the causal chain.

Using sensitive laboratory technologies, biomarkers of exposure can detect low levels of exposure. Although these biomarkers are usually designed to measure the exposure of environmental toxicants, they can also identify levels of ingested dietary components, bacterial and viral infections, and serve as endpoints in the determination of the success of intervention strategies. Thus, there are 2 types of biomarkers of exposure. The first one is the quantitative measurement of a chemical or its metabolite in human tissues, excretions, and/ or exhaled air. Examples are mercury in fingernails and toenails that provides direct measurements of exposure to mercury; hippuric acid in urine and toluene in blood as biomarkers of exposure to toluene; tobacco-specific nitrosamines as a biomarker of tobacco exposure. The second type is the measurement of an early reversible biochemical change in a biological fluid that reflects exposure, such as measurements of sucrose and fructose in 24-hour urine samples to directly assess sugar consumption, or "concentration" of biomarkers, such as urine 3-(3,5-dihydroxyphenyl)-1-propanoic acid (DHPPA), which are related to whole-grain wheat and rye intake but only indirectly because their levels are the result of complex metabolic processes.

Biomarkers of exposure must be evaluated in terms of their ability to predict and quantify exposure. Certain properties are desirable when linking a biomarker with exposure.

①The biomarker should be specific to environmental toxicants, ingested dietary components, bacterial or viral infections, which is of primary interest. For example, the urinary aflatoxin-DNA adduct is a specific measure for dietary aflatoxin contamination.

②The biomarker should remain long enough in the body to make sure its measurement is reliable. Nicotine is the most abundant alkaloid found in the tobacco leaf. The plasma nicotine level is effective for assessing nicotine intake and its pharmacologic effects within a narrow window of exposure; however, it is not ideal for monitoring tobacco exposure over extended periods due to its short half-life (two hours). In contrast, blood, salivary or urinary cotinine, a metabolite of nicotine, is more advantageous as a tobacco biomarker due to its long elimination time and half-life (16—18 hours).

③The biomarker should present in an accessible tissue—for example, be present in urine, blood, or saliva.

④The biomarker should be able to detect low levels of exposure and classify individuals based on their exposure status.

⑤The biomarker should be relatively inexpensive to measure in many samples.

⑥The biomarker should be of value in establishing the biological plausibility of an exposure-disease association.

Exposure biomarkers are widely used because they can provide information on the route, absorbed dose, pathway, and sometimes, even the source of exposure. These indicators also allow researchers to work forward in time to determine an exposure and prevent it from causing further damage. The elevated level of an exposure biomarker should be removed if the individual ceases or reduces the exposure.

11.2.3   Effect Biomarkers

An effect biomarker is a quantifiable change that an individual endures, indicating potential adverse effects of a chemical on a physiological process or organ system. Examples are (a) retinol binding protein in urine as effect biomarkers of heavy metals such as cadmium exposure; (b) elevated aminotransferase enzymes in serum as biomarkers of liver injury from carbon tetrachloride exposure; and (c) the presence of DNA adducts, micronuclei, and chromosomal aberrations in peripheral lymphocytes as biomarkers of possible genotoxic effects from exposure to polyaromatic hydrocarbons and aromatic amines.

Effect biomarkers indicating a preclinical response are not always detectable using conventional clinical diagnostic tools. Individuals show elevated levels of effect biomarkers before the onset of overt disease. In some cases, after removal of exposure, the effect biomarker, once expressed, may not return to normal.

A disadvantage of most effect biomarkers is that they generally are no-specific for a single chemical, but reflecting cumulative exposure to a variety of environmental factors or even the endogenous metabolism process. As shown in Table 11.1, most effect biomarkers cannot be used to assess exposure to a specific chemical.

11.2.4   Susceptibility Biomarkers

A susceptibility biomarker is an indicator of an inherent or acquired ability of the target subject to respond adversely to a given environmental agent. In other words, a susceptibility biomarker is a biomarker that is associated with an increased or decreased chance of developing a disease or medical condition in an individual who, from a clinical standpoint, does not yet have that disease or medical condition. Susceptibility biomarkers may be detectable many years—in some cases decades-before the appearance of clinical signs and symptoms.

One of the major risk factors for colorectal cancer is family history, and approximately 20% of colorectal cancer patients report a history of the disease among first- or second-degree relatives. Genes responsible for inherited colorectal cancer have been identified; such as the $MLH1$ and $MSH2$ genes involved in the DNA repair pathway, and tumor suppressor gene APC. In addition, by genotyping colorectal cancer patients from epidemiologic studies, researchers showed that polymorphisms in methylenetetrahydrofolate reductase ($MTHFR$), glutathione S-transferase M1 ($GSTM1$), and glutathione S-transferase T1 ($GSTT1$) are associated with colorectal cancer risk.

Another familiar example of a susceptibility biomarker is the breast cancer genes 1 and 2 ($BRCA1/2$) mutations. Researchers found that changes in these two genes could help identify individuals with a predisposition to developing breast cancer. However, having these high-risk mutation does not mean that a woman will definitely develop breast cancer. The main utility of susceptibility biomarkers in clinical practice is to guide prevention. In May 2013, Angelina Jolie, a world-famous actress, had "preventative surgery" to remove both breasts after discovering that she carries $BRCA1$ mutations.

11.3　Research Methods

11.3.1　Research Design and Analysis

In general, descriptive epidemiology, analytical epidemiology and experimental epidemiology can be applied in molecular epidemiology studies, and researchers can adopt different study designs according to different research purposes. However, descriptive studies and prospective cohort studies require considerable sample sizes, and molecular biology experiments for biomarkers detection are expensive, as a result, case-control studies are widely used.

11.3.1.1　Case-Control Study

The design of a case-control study of molecular epidemiology does not differ substantially from the design of a traditional case-control study. Taking the study of genetic polymorphism and genetic susceptibility as an example, controls should be selected from the population that gives rise to the study cases. A "false positive" result can be achieved if cases come from a population with a high frequency of polymorphism, controls are selected from a population with a low frequency of polymorphism. We should gather data preferably from incident rather than prevalent cases; Otherwise, it will cause the prevalence-incidence bias. Case-Control studies are suitable for studies of genetic variants. Unlike other biologic markers of exposures such as hormonal levels and DNA adducts, genetic markers are stable indicators of host susceptibility. Additionally, case-control studies can organize a comprehensive search for the effects of several genes, along with other possible risk factors, and explore the effects of gene-environment interaction on the development of the disease. However, in the molecular epidemiology of cancer and other chronic diseases, in which a biomarker is measured, the case-control study is limited if the marker has a short half-life, i. e. it refers to exposures that took place a short time before the disease onset.

11.3.1.2   Nested Case-Control Study

This study is essentially a case-control study based on a cohort study. In the nested case-control study, cases that occur in a defined cohort are identified and, for each, a specified number of matched controls are selected from among those in the cohort who have not developed the disease by the time of disease occurrence in the case. In other words, the cases and controls come from the same cohort. Since exposure information and biological samples have been collected during the baseline investigation, selection bias and information bias can be avoided, making the subjects more representative and comparable. In general, the most promising design for future studies of molecular epidemiology is certainly the nested case-control study.

11.3.1.3   Case-Only Study

In case-control studies, it is difficult to choose appropriate controls, especially in molecular epidemiology studies. Obtaining biological samples from healthy controls is also restricted by medical ethics. The basic feature of case-only studies is that the only case is used as the subject, which avoids the selection bias caused by the selection of controls. The basic principle is to process the data of cases with different clinical types or with some biological markers and those without biological markers according to the way of a case-control study, to explore the difference of risk factors of different clinical types or the relationship and interaction between this biological marker and other risk factors of the disease. The case-only study has received huge attention due to its potential use in the investigation of gene-gene and gene-environment interactions. The design may be especially useful for rare diseases because the sample sizes required to detect the interaction between two genes, or between genes and environmental exposures, are smaller for the case-only design than the case-control design and other designs.

11.3.1.4   Linkage Analysis

Linkage analysis is an important epidemiological analysis method that carries out genotyping in family member samples and uses the genetic statistical analysis method to determine the genetic mode and transmission rule of heredity related diseases and identify the phenotype related genes or regions by drawing the genetic relation map. Linkage analysis is the predominant statistical genetic mapping approach used in the latter half of the twentieth century. In the early stage, it was mainly applied to the identification of genetic defects in patients with single-gene genetic diseases. More recently, the focus shifts to association studies of complex traits that analyze common variants. However, for such variants, genome-wide association studies (GWASs) are more powerful than linkage analyses. Recently, it has been suggested that rare variation has a stronger influence on disease susceptibility. With the development of the new generation of sequencing technology, the research design of linkage analysis has received new attention due to the unique advantages of family-based design in the analysis of rare variation.

11.3.2　Collection and Storage of Biological Samples

11.3.2.1　Biological Specimen Bank

Molecular epidemiology needs to obtain information from biological specimens, which generally include pathogenic specimens and biological specimens of the human body. The collection process should be carried out following standard operating procedures. Biological specimens are stored in the biological specimen bank according to standard procedures, and the corresponding specimens should be selected for index detection according to the research content. Biological specimen bank is a system that stores one or more types of biological specimens and maintains their biological activity, such as serum bank, tissue bank, pathogenic microorganism bank and so on. The key points of the establishment of biological specimen bank are ①Biological specimens cannot be contaminated during collection and storage; ②Stable and consistent results can be obtained when the stored biological specimens are tested within the effective time; ③All biological specimens should have detailed background material and identification.

11.3.2.2　Biological Specimens in Molecular Epidemiology Study

Common biological specimens include blood specimens (red blood cells, white blood cells, plasma or serum), tissue specimens and other specimens (saliva, urine, hair, semen, gastric juice, etc.). The following is a brief introduction to common biological specimens in molecular epidemiological studies.

Blood can be centrifuged to collect red blood cells (RBCs), white blood cells (WBCs), plasma or serum. RBC is a source of hemoglobin which can be used for the measurement of adducts. In general, WBC is a source of genomic DNA that can be used, for example, for the genotyping of subjects. Serum or plasma can be used to detect levels of nutrients, hormones, non-coding RNA, and other biomarkers.

Oral buccal cells can be used to extract genomic DNA instead of blood, and the sample source is easy, non-invasive, simple and fast. However, because of the low DNA content, it is not suitable for the detection of high requirements on DNA content.

Urine can be used to detect a variety of biomarkers associated with exposure and metabolism.

Hair can be used to detect chemicals, i. e. arsenic.

(1) The Goals of Collection Procedures:

①In the molecular epidemiology studies, the corresponding biomarkers should be selected according to the different research purposes.

②The number of biological specimens should be reasonable, not too much or too little.

③To avoid contamination of specimens. For example, urine is not mixed with other body fluids such as menstrual blood.

④To ensure the correction of the anticoagulant type and anticoagulant ratio.

⑤To ensure the labels are clear and correct, including sample number, sampling time, etc.

⑥To ensure the collection of biological material in ways that are acceptable to subjects.

(2)The Goals of Storage Procedures

①To ensure optimal preservation of biological specimens. At -20℃, urine is stable; At -70℃, cell viability (if not cryopreserved) is limited although DNA, serum and most hormones are stable.

②To avoid the quality of specimens affected by long storage time.

③To ensure easy matching of biological specimens with individual identity.

④Ethics should be followed in the whole process of specimen management to protect the privacy of the subject.

(3)Detection Methods of Biomarkers

After a preliminary selection of biomarkers, it is necessary to select appropriate methods for detection. The detection methods of biomarkers are divided into molecular biology technology, serology technology and immunology technology, and the most widely used one is the molecular biology technologies, such as nucleic acid research technology, protein research technology, enzyme technology and biochip technology. Genetic variation in genes, such as single nucleotide polymorphisms (SNPs), is often detected in molecular epidemiological studies. Common genotyping techniques include TaqMan, SNPstream and OpenArray. Various high-throughput genotyping platforms based on chip technology and second-generation sequencing technology have also been widely used.

(4)Analysis of the Association Between Gene Polymorphism and Disease

By analyzing the differences in the allele distributions and genotype frequencies between cases and controls, we can determine the association between gene polymorphism and disease risk. Dominant model, recessive model, codominant model, overdominant model, and additive model can be used to estimate the relationship between different alleles and phenotypes. Assuming A is the reference allele and B is the variant allele, so AA is homozygous wild, AB is heterozygous and BB is homozygous mutational. The dominant model is AB/BB *vs* AA, the recessive model is BB *vs* AA/AB, the codominant model is AB *vs* AA and BB *vs* AA, the overdominant model is AA/BB *vs* AB, and the additive model is to assess the effect of the Increase in the number of B mutant alleles on the phenotype.

11.3.3   Ethical Issues in Biomarker Research

Application of biomarkers in epidemiological studies may raise ethical issues and social implications during protocol development, recruitment of participants, informed consent, and the interpretation and notification of study results. In addition, there are ethical considerations related to the use of any type of biological specimens collected and stored for one research purpose and subsequently used for other purposes. A predominant ethical issue is the maintenance of subjects' privacy and the confidentiality of the test and study results. In particular, with the development of society, the internet has a huge and dual impression on the development of molecular genetics. In the era of big data, it is necessary to deal with the relationship between medical research data sharing needs and the protection for the privacy of subjects. Consequently, each study must be approved by the ethics committee. Ethics committees need to have adequate knowledge of the purpose, scope and limitations of biomarker research to be able to correctly deal with the use of biomarkers in molecular epidemiology studies.

Beauchamp and Childress proposed four principles in their book, *Principles of Biomedical Ethics*. They are ① respect for patient autonomy; ② beneficence; ③ nonmaleficence; and ④ justice. The perspective of these principles has become the major approach to medical ethics in the last couple of decades. In addition to these four principles, the following requirements should be met when creating a database for molecular epidemiology (source: William W. Lowrance. "The Promise of Human Genetic Databases"):

①Following respectful protocols in obtaining information.

②Securing broad informed consent, for example, the commercial application of tests and study results.

③Managing anonymization of database interlinking and other privacy issues.

④Establishing confidentiality and security safeguards.

⑤Developing defensible responses to requests for personal data by various parties.

⑥Devising sound data access, ownership, and intellectual property policies.

⑦Being clear about whether and how individuals will be informed of findings that might be medically helpful for them.

⑧Arranging supervision by research ethics and privacy protection bodies.

11.4　Applications and Outlook

Since the 1980s, the necessity of using biomarkers as surrogate outcomes in large trials of major diseases, such as cancer and heart disease, has been widely discussed. Technological advances continue to produce innovative molecular biological techniques. Biomarker groups expanded from DNA adducts, epigenetic markers, RNA-based markers, to gene mutations and "omic" studies (transcriptomics, proteomics, and metabolomics). Biomarkers provide a dynamic and powerful approach to understand the spectrum of disease with applications in observational and analytic epidemiology, and randomized clinical trials. Defined as alterations in the constituents of tissues or body fluids, these markers offer the means for homogeneous classification of a disease and risk factors, and they can extend our base information about the underlying pathogenesis of the disease. Biomarkers can also reflect the entire spectrum of disease from the earliest manifestations to the terminal stages.

In epidemiological investigations, biomarkers improve validity while reducing bias in the measurement of exposures for the disease. Rather than relying on a history of exposure to a putative risk factor, direct measurement of the exposure or gene-environment interaction lessens the possibility of misclassification of exposure. Such misclassifications not only produce inaccurate and deceptive results but also reduce the power of studies. Thus, the use of biomarkers improves the sensitivity and specificity of the measurement of the exposures or risk factors.

Biomarkers of exposure can provide far more, however, to the field of disease epidemiology than the improvement of the exposure metric. For example, such biomarkers are also of value in establishing the biological plausibility of an association between a risk factor and disease. If a particular chemical exposure from ambient air is associated with increased risk, the additional information that exposed individuals have higher levels of DNA damage would add support to the exposure-disease association. Alternatively, if a particular genetic polymorphism associated with increased cardiovascular risk is also linked to higher levels of a biomarker on the presumed causal pathway, e. g. , atherosclerosis, then this would provide support for the original association. These types of mechanistic data are increasingly considered in the processes of hazard identification and cancer or cardiovascular disease risk assessment.

Biomarkers can also help evaluate the dose-effect and sometimes more accurately dose-response relationships by describing and quantifying the relationship between exposure or absorbed dose and related health outcomes. Often this component of the assessment is hindered by the lack of appropriate methods necessary to extrapolate data from high-dose (e. g. , occupational exposure settings) to low-dose exposure (e. g. , general air pollution exposure conditions) or from animal models to humans.

Biomarkers depicting prodromal signs enable earlier diagnosis or allow for the outcome of interest to be determined at a more primitive stage of the disease. In these conditions, biomarkers are used as an indicator of a biological factor that represents either a subclinical manifestation, stage of the disorder, or a surrogate manifestation of the disease.

High-risk groups are important to be identified in epidemiology, particularly concerning environmental health hazards. Since individuals have varied exposures and susceptibility, the standards for protective measures should be set based on the most vulnerable population groups, that is, public health policies should attempt to provide protective measures to those who are most susceptible. Meanwhile, the potential uses of this class of biomarkers include: ① Reduction in disease heterogeneity in clinical trials or epidemiologic studies or outcome indicators of clinical trials. For example, triple-negative breast cancers were defined as those that were estrogen receptor-negative, progesterone receptor-negative, and HER2/neu-negative. Triple-negative breast cancers were found to have a more aggressive clinical course than other forms of breast cancer. ② Target for a clinical trial. The use of biomarkers is easier and less expensive than direct measurement of the clinical endpoint, and biomarkers are usually measured over a shorter period. The FDA continues to promote the use of biomarkers in basic and clinical research, as well as research on potential new biomarkers to use as surrogates in future trials.

Another valuable application of biomarkers is to evaluate the potential value of intervention strategies. This may be primary prevention to reduce exposure, or more mechanism-based approaches such as chemoprevention. For example, lung cancer patients harboring mutations in the epidermal growth factor receptor ($EGFR$) would respond to $EGFR$ tyrosine kinase inhibitors.

The rapid growth of molecular biology and laboratory technology has expanded to the point at which the application of technically advanced biomarkers will soon become even more feasible. Molecular biomarkers will, in the hands of clinical investigators, provide a dynamic and powerful approach to understand the spectrum of disease with obvious applications in analytical epidemiology, clinical trials and disease prevention, diagnosis, and disease management.

(Yu Qiong, Yin Jieyun, Wang Hui, Zhao Jinshun)

Exercise

Chapter 12　Systematic Review and Meta-Analysis

Evidence-based medicine (EBM), defined as the "integration of best research evidence with clinical expertise and patient values", has been gaining popularity in the past decade. EBM aims to optimize decision-making by emphasizing the use of best evidence from well-designed and -conducted research. It is a revolutionary reform in medical practice of the 21st century and has a great influence on the research and practice of clinical medicine. The theory has been applied to many aspects of health services, such as medical practices, nursing, prevention, and medical education. As EBM continues to develop, systematic reviews have become the standard method to evaluate and synthesize research results and provide evidence for decision-making. This chapter introduces the concept of systematic review and meta-analysis and describes how these methodologies should be conducted.

12. 1　Introduction to Systematic Review

12. 1. 1　Basic Concept of Systematic Review

Systematic review is an approach to literature reviews that was proposed by Archie Cochrane in 1979. A systematic review is essentially a structured investigation of existing research data identified via a reproducible standardized search leading to data abstraction, appraisal of methodological quality, clinical relevance, and consistency of published evidence on a specific clinical topic to provide clear suggestions for a specific health care problem. Studies used for systematic review can be of interventions (i. e. , randomized controlled trials) or observations (i. e. , case-control or cohort studies). The type of study included depends on the investigator's research question. Results from systematic reviews are used to formulate research questions that are narrow in scope. Using systematic reviews, researchers can identify and synthesize studies that directly relate to the systematic review question and provide a complete, exhaustive summary of current evidence relevant to a research question. Systematic reviews of randomized controlled trials are key to the practice of EBM, and a review of existing studies is often quicker and cheaper than embarking on a new study. In addition to assessing clinical treatments, systematic reviews also concern disease etiology, diagnostic tests, prognosis, and public health interventions.

Good systematic reviews have several strengths: ① Comprehensive search strategy. Good systematic reviews usually scan multiple sources of information, such as using electronic databases or specialized registers of trials, hand searching, expert consultation, and personal contacts to retrieve relevant studies. ②Explicit methodology. Systematic reviews are undertaken on the premise that they should be reproducible like any other scientific activity. This requires that the methods to conduct the review should be described in such detail that allows any other reviewer to reproduce it with the same results. A proper systematic review contains a "methods" section to explicitly describe the steps and definitions used. ③Emphasis on all clinically important outcomes. Systematic reviews emphasize all clinically relevant outcomes related to the efficacy, safety, and tolerability of the interventions under considerations. ④Limiting errors. Systematic reviews usually have two reviewers at all major steps to limit errors in conducting the review. Reviewers appraise the quality and quantity of data and give appropriate weights to the studies under review. This tends to limit bias and improve prediction value in what to expect while extrapolating the results.

12. 1. 2　Classification of Systematic Review

When the results of primary studies are summarized but not statistically combined, the review may be called a qualitative systematic review. A quantitative systematic review, or meta-analysis, is a systematic review that uses statistical methods to combine the results of two or more studies. The term overview is sometimes used to denote a systematic review, whether it is quantitative or qualitative. Summaries of research that lack explicit descriptions of systematic methods are often called narrative reviews.

12. 1. 3　Differences Between Systematic Review and Traditional Review

The purpose of a literature review is to provide summary information that helps the reader understand a particular topic without having to read all the published materials on this topic. Literature reviews consist of systematic review and traditional review (or narrative review). Traditional review may involve multiple aspects of one specific problem (e. g. , pathology, pathophysiology, diagnosis, prevention, and treatment or rehabilitation of hypertension) or only one aspect of this problem (e. g. , treatment). In contrast, systematic reviews focus on a specific aspect of a clinical problem and deal with it formally and in depth. Thus, a narrative review is helpful for understanding the whole picture of a disease, while a systematic review will address particular aspects of a disease, such as the optimal methods of diagnosis or treatment. The main differences between the two are shown in Table 12. 1.

Table 12. 1　Differences Between a Systematic Review and a Traditional Review

Feature	Systematic Review	Traditional Review
Review question	Focused, well-defined clinical question formulated with PICO framework	Question is usually broad and not well defined
Protocol	A priori protocol is developed and published	No protocol

(To be continued)

Table 12. 1

Feature	Systematic Review	Traditional Review
Methods	Usually very well-defined and explicitly stated with study inclusion and exclusion criteria	Usually not well-defined
Literature search	A good systematic review includes a well-defined comprehensive search, without language or other restrictions	Search strategy is usually not stated, and the review is confined to well-known articles often supporting the authors' views
Critical appraisal	Internal validity of the individual studies included in a systematic review is vetted by various tools such as the Cochrane risk of bias assessment tool	Critical appraisal is usually not performed
Synthesis	Qualitative (sometimes quantitative with meta-analysis); may answer a clinical question unanswerable by individual studies	Usually qualitative summary
Findings/conclusion	Findings are reproducible	Findings are not reproducible. Author's personal belief may influence the overall conclusion of a traditional review

12. 2   Essential Steps of Systematic Review

12. 2. 1   Research Question and Protocol

Systematic review, like any other research activity, starts with a research question. The research question specifies the population of interest, the exposure or intervention, the comparison (in certain situations) and the outcome of interest. This principle of formatting research problems is called **PICO**, which can, ultimately, establish the research question.

- Patient/Person: to whom does this relate?
- Intervention (or cause, prognosis): what is the intervention or cause?
- Comparison: to what can the intervention be compared?
- Outcome: in what outcomes you are interested?

This PICO format is used as a guide to ensure that all topics required to answer the question have been covered. For example, the PICO format for the question of "does Tamiflu help to prevent the flu" would be:

- P: people with the flu
- I: Tamiflu
- C: without using Tamiflu
- O: reduction in flu symptoms and/or duration

This may require several revisions, and some scoping of the literature to identify a question that is specific and answerable. A clear, specific, and answerable question is essential to a successful review.

The protocol is important and must specify the research question, search methods, criteria for including or excluding a study, criteria for quality assessment (appraisal) of the studies and methods of data extraction and synthesis. Subgroup analyses, if any, are pre-specified. Cochrane (previously known as the Cochrane Collaboration) developed a system of reviewing the protocol and publishing it in the Cochrane Library. The steps detailed below are then followed according to the protocol. To avoid wasting time and energy, we should establish whether this question has already been answered in the published literature, or is registered as an ongoing review (e. g. , search in DARE, which contains abstracts of quality assessed systematic reviews and details of all Cochrane reviews and protocols).

12. 2. 2 Comprehensive Search

This can be complex and requires searching in different databases (different reviews require different search strategies) as well as locating non-published studies, e. g. , by contacting experts in the field, or hand-searching conference proceedings. One conclusion seems clear from empirical studies—no single source is comprehensive enough. Reviewers adopt multiple overlapping methods to ascertain the relevant studies as comprehensively as possible. MEDLINE, arguably the most popular source for medical literature, does not yield all the relevant studies and what it yields is often irrelevant. Non-MEDLINE electronic databases (Embase, Cochrane Library, PubMed, etc.) should also be searched. Cochrane review groups have searched coordinators to maintain a specialized register of studies and found relevant ones. Reviewers display posters with a list of studies in conferences and seek additional studies from subject experts. The experts often point to additional studies (published as well as unpublished). Writing to the experts can also be rewarding in this regard; for example, many reviewers write to drug manufacturers to gather unpublished studies of a drug.

12. 2. 3 Selection of Studies

Reviewers use predefined inclusion (and exclusion) criteria to select studies for review. The criteria refer to the study design, specific population, intervention, comparison, and outcome relevant for the research question based on the PICO. Studies meeting the criteria are selected for the next steps. Usually, by screening the title and/or the abstract, many of the papers identified will be rejected, because they do not fulfil the inclusion criteria. The investigator should then generate a "long-list" of all the papers required for further, more detailed reading (erring on the side of over-inclusion). These papers may be retrieved from the library or e-journals, by copying the paper original or requesting an inter-library loan. The researcher should keep a record of why he or she rejected each one so that the PRISMA flowchart may be completed. Ideally, this should be done by two researchers independently (it is very easy to miss one or two articles when screening large numbers), and disputes can be settled between them or through a discussion with a third person.

12. 2. 4　Data Extraction

One of the most important and time-consuming parts of a systematic review is data extraction. Data is extracted independently by two reviewers and any disagreements are resolved by discussion or arbitration by a third reviewer. Table 12. 2 summarizes the key information that should be extracted. Each review question is unique and therefore requires the development of a separate form. A pilot electronic or paper version of the data extraction form includes entries for study characteristics along with relevant results and risk of bias assessment. The data extraction form should first be piloted on two to three studies.

Table 12. 2　Information to Consider in Data Extraction Form

Data Extraction	Information to Consider in Data Extraction
Reviewer identification	Review author ID; date
Study identification	Study ID; report ID; citation; author contact details; publication year; country; source of data
Methods	Study design; setting; enrolment period; no. of centers
Participant characteristics	Total number; age; sex; co-morbidity; ethnicity; number of lost to follow-up
Disease characteristics	Staging; severity; biological behavior; surgical complexity; method of diagnosis
Interventions[a]	Surgical technique; surgeon experience/volume; drug dose, route of delivery and length
Diagnostic test characteristics[b]	Description of the reference standard, index test, comparator, manufacturer; interpreter of diagnostic test
Prognostic factor characteristics[c]	Dose, level, duration of exposure; method of measurement
Outcome	Outcome definition (including unit of measurement, scale, assessor, time point of measurement)
Results to include in a meta-analysis	Dichotomous outcomes: no. of events/no. of participants Continuous outcomes: mean value and SD in each intervention group Time-to-event outcomes: HR (with 95% CI) Diagnostic test performance outcomes: TP, FP, TN, FN
Risk of bias	Cochrane risk of bias tool for RCTs or other tools such as QUIPS and QUADAS-2
Other	Review author comments

CI=confidence interval; FN=false negative; FP=false positive; HR=hazard ratio; ID=identification; RCT=randomized controlled trial; SD=standard deviation; TN=true negative; TP=true positive.

[a] For comparative effectiveness of interventions systematic reviews.

[b] For diagnostic test accuracy systematic reviews.

[c] For prognostic factor systematic reviews.

The setting and timing of the study, participants, and disease characteristics (such as age, sex, comorbidities, diagnostic criteria, staging, and prognostic factors) that may influence intervention effects or external validity should be collected. Relevant information includes surgical techniques, drug doses and frequency, or routes of delivery. It is important to decide the outcome measures that will be collected in terms of their definition (e. g. , measurement method, scale, and threshold), timing, and unit(s) of measurement. This is crucial because many outcomes may be reported using multiple definitions (e. g. , biochemical recurrence after radical prostatectomy), measurement scales (e. g. , multiple urinary symptom questionnaires to access the severity of urinary incontinence), measurement method (e. g. , healthy parenchymal volume loss after partial nephrectomy measured by computed tomography volumetric analysis or estimated by surgeon), or different points in time. Standardized sets of outcomes, known as "core outcome sets", represent the minimum that should be measured and reported in all clinical trials of a specific condition making it easier for the results of trials to be combined. The numerical data required for the meta-analysis is not always available and sometimes other statistics or graphical information can be collected and converted into the required format.

12. 2. 5   Risk of Bias Assessment

Bias can lead to either an overestimation or an underestimation of the effect of an intervention, resulting in heterogeneity between study outcomes. No consensus currently exists regarding the best way to assess the risk of bias (RoB), but most methods are based on the study design. For example, Cochrane's RoB Tool is used for RCTs. QUADAS-2 is used for assessing RoB in diagnostic test accuracy systematic reviews, while QUIPS is used for prognostic factor systematic reviews.

12. 2. 5. 1   RCTs

In RCT systematic reviews, the RoB in each study is assessed for each outcome using the domains (judged as either low, high, or unclear) in the Cochrane RoB Tool:

• Selection bias, which includes random sequence generation bias and allocation of concealment bias.

• Performance bias due to the knowledge of the allocated intervention by study personnel and participants.

• Detection bias in assessing the outcome due to the knowledge of the allocated intervention.

• Attrition bias due to incomplete data and exclusion from analyses.

• Reporting bias due to selective outcome reporting.

• Other sources of bias.

RevMan is then used to create an RoB summary graph to visually illustrate the RoB (low, high, or unclear) for each domain in each study.

12. 2. 5. 2   Nonrandomized Comparative Studies

Potential biases are greater in nonrandomized comparative studies (NRCSs) than in

RCTs due to the high risk of confounding. As a result, NRCSs are always considered to be at high risk of selection bias. In addition to assessing the above domains for RCTs, a maximum of the five most important confounders should be prespecified. For each outcome, an assessment is made of ①whether the confounder was considered, ②whether its distribution was balanced, and if not, ③whether it was controlled in the analysis. This information is used to reach an overall decision about the RoB for each confounder and each outcome. The RoB summary graph can also include additional confounder information. Recently, ROB-INS-I, a tool for assessing the risk of bias in nonrandomized studies of interventions has been published.

12. 2. 5. 3   Single Arm Studies

In systematic reviews of single-arm case series, five aspects are considered: ① Was there a priori protocol? ②Was the total population included or were study participants selected consecutively? ③Was outcome data complete for all participants and any missing data adequately explained/unlikely to be related to the outcome? ④ Were all prespecified outcomes of interest and expected outcomes reported? ⑤ Were primary benefit and harm outcomes appropriately measured? If the answer to all five questions is "yes", the study is at "low" RoB. If the answer to any question is "no", the study is at a "high" RoB.

12. 2. 5. 4   RoB Assessment Process

Two reviewers independently assess the RoB in each study when extracting data. A third reviewer acts as an arbitrator. If the RoB is unclear in any domain, an attempt is made to obtain the study protocol or to contact the study authors. RoB summary graphs are created with separate graphs for each of the three different study types. Biases are described in the systematic review report, emphasizing areas of concern and the possible effect of bias in interpreting the results.

12. 2. 6   Data Synthesis

The data from the studies can be presented narratively and/or statistically (a meta-analysis). If studies are significantly heterogenous, it may be most appropriate to summarize the data narratively and not attempt a statistical (meta-analytic) summary.

All systematic reviews should contain text and tables to provide an initial descriptive summary and explanation of the characteristics and findings of the included studies. However, simply describing the studies is not sufficient for a synthesis. The defining characteristic of narrative synthesis is the adoption of a textual approach that provides an analysis of the relationships within and between studies and an overall assessment of the robustness of the evidence. Narrative synthesis is inherently a more subjective process than meta-analysis; therefore, the approach should be rigorous and transparent enough to reduce the potential for bias. The idea of narrative synthesis within a systematic review should not be confused with broader terms like "narrative review", which are sometimes used to describe reviews that are not systematic.

How narrative syntheses are carried out varies widely, and historically there has been a lack of consensus as to the constituent elements of the approach or the conditions for establishing credibility. A project for the Economic and Social Research Council (ESRC) Method Program has developed guidance for conducting narrative synthesis in systematic reviews. The guidance offers both a general framework and specific tools and techniques that help to increase the transparency and trustworthiness of narrative synthesis. The general framework consists of four elements: ①Developing a theory of how the intervention works, why, and for whom; ②Developing a preliminary synthesis of findings of included studies; ③Exploring relationships within and between studies; ④Assessing the robustness of the synthesis.

A statistical synthesis should include numerical and graphical presentations of the data, and also look at the strength and consistency of the evidence and investigate reasons for any inconsistencies (See Section 12.3 on meta-analysis).

12.2.7　Presenting Results

It is essential that systematic review be presented clearly using current best practices. The PRISMA statement and related articles provide very clear guidance on reporting systematic reviews, including a flow chart of studies included. Report writing is an integral part of the systematic review process. This section deals with the primary scientific report of the review, which often takes the form of a comprehensive report to the commissioning body. The report should describe the review methods clearly and in sufficient detail that others could repeat them, if they wished. Evidence suggests that the quality of reporting in primary studies may affect the readers' interpretation of the results, and the same is likely to be true of systematic reviews. It has also been argued that trials and reviews often provide incomplete or omit the crucial "how-to" details about interventions, limiting a clinicians' ability to implement findings in practice.

12.2.8　Update the Systematic Review

Updating systematic reviews is, in general, more efficient than starting afresh when new evidence emerges. The panel for updating guidance for systematic reviews met to develop guidance for people considering updating systematic reviews. Decisions about whether and when to update a systematic review are judgments made for individual reviews at a particular time. These decisions can be made by agencies responsible for systematic review portfolios, journal editors with systematic review update services, or author teams considering embarking on an update of a review. The decision must consider whether the review addresses a current question, uses valid methods, and is well conducted; and whether new relevant methods, new studies, or new information on existing studies are included. Given this information, the agency, editors, or authors must judge whether the update will influence the review findings or credibility sufficiently to justify the effort in updating it. Search strategies should be refined, considering changes in the question or inclusion criteria. An analysis of yield from the previous edition, databases, terms, and languages can make searches more specific and efficient. In many instances, an update represents a new edition of the review, and authorship of the new version needs to follow the criteria of the International Committee of Medical Journal Editors (ICMJE). New approaches to publishing licenses could help new authors build on and re-use the previous edition while giving appropriate credit to the previous authors.

12.3　Introduction to Meta-Analysis

12.3.1　What Is Meta-Analysis?

Simply stated, a meta-analysis is a study of studies. The National Library of Medicine (NLM) defines meta-analysis as a "quantitative method of combining the results of independent studies (usually drawn from the published literature) and synthesizing summaries and conclusions which may be used to evaluate therapeutic effectiveness, plan new studies, etc., with application chiefly in the areas of research and medicine". Meta-analyses are often, but not always, important components of a systematic review procedure. A systematic review may have only qualitative or both qualitative and quantitative components; the qualitative component consists of the assessment of the quality of individual studies, whereas the quantitative component is the meta-analysis.

12.3.2　Basic Process of Meta-Analysis

12.3.2.1　Formulation of the Research Question

A meta-analysis starts with a research question. The research question specifies the "PICO" model: the patients or population of interest, the intervention or exposure, the comparison (in certain situations), and the outcome of interest. (The reader may refer to the similar research question formulation in the systematic review.)

12.3.2.2　Searching for Studies

Once the question is well formulated, the researcher must find the current best evidence to answer the question. The principle of searching for studies to find the current best evidence is a comprehensive search that maximizes the collection of all studies related to the research question. There is no way to prove that a reviewer has found all the relevant studies, but the fact remains clear that no single source is comprehensive enough.

12.3.2.3　Selection of Studies

Reviewers select studies based on predefined explicit incorporation criteria (inclusion criteria) and exclusion criteria. The criteria refer to the specific subjects, study designs, interventions, outcomes related to the research question, sample sizes, observation period, time of publication, publication types, and languages, etc.

A typical process for selecting meta-analysis studies is as follows:

①Merging search results using reference management software and removing duplicate records of the same report.

②Examining titles and abstracts to remove irrelevant reports (authors should generally be over-inclusive at this stage).

③Retrieving full text of the potentially relevant reports.

④Linking multiple reports of the same study.

⑤Examining full-text reports for compliance of studies with eligibility criteria.

⑥Corresponding with investigators, where appropriate, to clarify study eligibility (it may be appropriate to request further information, such as missing results, at the same time).

⑦Making final decisions on study inclusion and proceeding to data collection.

12.3.2.4 Quality Assessment of Studies

The extent to which a meta-analysis can draw the right conclusion about the effects of an intervention depends on whether the data and results from the included studies are valid. The quality assessment of the validity of the included studies is an essential component of a meta-analysis as well as a Cochrane review. An assessment of a study's validity should emphasize the risk of bias (e. g. , selection bias, performance bias, attrition bias, detection bias, and reporting bias) that will overestimate or underestimate the true intervention effect, and the criteria to assess the included studies, which may include the basic elements of credibility of randomization, blinded outcome assessment, extent of follow-up, and intention-to-treat analysis.

12.3.2.5 Data Collection and Extraction

In this section, we define "data" as any information about (or deriving from) a study, including details of methods, basic study design characteristics, participants, setting, context, interventions, outcome measures, results, publications, and investigators. Raw data on unpublished or negative results can also be obtained from the authors of original studies if necessary. In any case, reviewers should plan what data will be required for their meta-analysis and formulate a strategy to obtain them.

12.3.2.6 Data Analysis

Data analysis is one of the most important steps in a meta-analysis. There are five sub-steps: ①Assessing combinability; ②Selecting the formula for combining; ③Weighting the studies in a meta-analysis; ④Combining results on benefits, risks, and tolerability; ⑤Analyzing the subgroup. For more details, see Section 12.3.5 General Approach to Pooling Data.

12. 3. 2. 7   Sensitivity Analysis

A sensitivity analysis aims to investigate the stability of the meta-analysis results. When researchers find evidence of a small effect, they should conduct sensitivity analyses to examine how the results of the meta-analysis change under different assumptions relating to the reasons for these effects. The following approaches of sensitivity analyses have been suggested: comparing estimates of fixed and random effects, trim and fill, stratifying studies according to quality, changing the inclusion and exclusion criteria, excluding poor-quality studies, or removing studies one by one, etc.

12. 3. 2. 8   Interpretation of Results

This is similar to the interpretation of a single study, except that a meta-analysis provides an opportunity to examine the consistency of the results across studies, across different subgroups of patients, across various outcome categories and about the quality of studies. The results section should summarize the findings in a clear, logical order and should explicitly address the objectives of the meta-analysis. Review authors can use a variety of tables and figures to present information in a more convenient format, including tables that describe the characteristics of included studies (including RoB tables), data and analyses (the full set of data tables and forest plots), figures (a selection of study flow diagrams, forest plots, funnel plots, RoB plots and other figures), tables that summarize findings, and additional tables. When heterogeneity is present among meta-analysis studies, the sources of heterogeneity and its effect on the size of the combined effects should be considered.

12. 3. 4   Heterogeneity

12. 3. 4. 1   What Is Heterogeneity?

The similarity of results of included studies in a meta-analysis is called "homogeneity". Dissimilarity is called "heterogeneity". Any kind of variability among studies in a meta-analysis may be termed heterogeneity. The types of heterogeneity are as follows.

①Clinical heterogeneity (also called clinical diversity): including the variability in the participants, interventions, comparisons, and outcome measurements.

②Methodological heterogeneity (sometimes called methodological diversity): including the variability in study design and RoB.

③Statistical heterogeneity: indicating the variability in the intervention effects being evaluated in the different studies. Statistical heterogeneity is a consequence of clinical or methodological diversity, or both, among the studies. Statistical heterogeneity manifests when the observed intervention effects vary more from each other than one would expect due to random error (chance) alone. We will follow convention and refer to statistical heterogeneity simply as heterogeneity.

12. 3. 4. 2　Identifying and Measuring Heterogeneity

The following five methods may be useful in identifying and measuring the heterogeneity of included studies.

①Examine the study design, study population, interventions, outcomes, and study methodology. Effects may differ depending on study designs because the degree of bias in the data differs from one design to another. Randomized controlled studies are generally less susceptible to bias than case-control studies. Similarly, effects may vary due to differences in the study population, type and dose of interventions and types of outcome measures and timing of their measurement. Also, whether the outcome measurement is blinded or open and whether randomization is concealed or unconcealed may make a difference in the results.

②Examine the point estimates in the forest plot. If they are close to each other, the results are likely to be similar.

③Examine whether the confidence intervals (usually 95%) overlap. If the lines representing the confidence intervals of the various studies in the forest plot overlap, this indicates that the results across the studies may be similar.

④Test homogeneity or heterogeneity. The above methods are based on clinical or common sense. A formal statistical test also exists, called the test of homogeneity (or, to use a simpler term, the test of similarity). This test asks the question: are the differences likely due to chance? The answer comes in the form of the P-value. If the P-value is over 0.10, the differences may be considered likely due to chance, and, if the study results are considered to be similar, then the researcher can use the fixed-effects model to calculate the size of the combined effect. If the P-value is less than 0.10, the researcher should explore the causes of heterogeneity among the study results. Heterogeneity may be explored by conducting subgroup analyses to investigate the characteristics of studies, such as study design, study population, intervention, outcomes and study methodology. If the results of the included studies are still heterogeneous after subgroup analysis, the researcher should choose the random-effects model to calculate the size of the combined effect.

It should be noted that the results of the test may sometimes be misleading. If the number and size of studies are small, the test may not pick up even important differences. On the other hand, if the number and size of studies are large, the test may overly highlight even small differences. The former situation is more common than the latter.

⑤Another statistic is I^2. This indicates the percentage of variability in effect estimates that is due to underlying differences in effect rather than chance. Formula (12.1) shows the way to calculate I^2:

$$I^2 = \left\{ \frac{Q-df}{Q} \right\} \times 100\% \tag{12.1}$$

where Q is the chi-squared statistic and df is its degrees of freedom. This describes the percentage of the variability in effect estimates that is due to heterogeneity rather than sampling error (chance).

Thresholds for the interpretation of I^2 can be misleading, since the importance of inconsistency depends on several factors. A rough guide to interpretation is as follows:

0%—40%: probably not important

30%—60%: may represent moderate heterogeneity *

50%—90%: may represent substantial heterogeneity *

75%—100%: considerable heterogeneity *

* The importance of the observed value of I^2 depends on ①magnitude and direction of effects and ②strength of evidence for heterogeneity (e. g. , P-value from the *chi-square* test, or a confidence interval for I^2).

12. 3. 4. 3   Addressing Heterogeneity

The following seven strategies may help address heterogeneity across the included studies for a meta-analysis.

①Check the data again.

②Do not pool the data if considerable variation exists in the results. In particular, if there is inconsistency in the direction of effect, it may be misleading to quote an average value for the intervention effect.

③Explore heterogeneity. Investigating characteristics of studies that may be associated with heterogeneity and conducting subgroup analyses or meta-regression may help in exploring heterogeneity.

④Ignore heterogeneity. Fixed-effect meta-analyses ignore heterogeneity.

⑤Perform a random-effects meta-analysis to incorporate heterogeneity among included studies.

⑥Change the effect measure.

⑦Exclude studies. One or two outlying studies with results that conflict with the rest of the studies may be the main cause of heterogeneity. If an obvious reason for the outlying result is apparent, the study might be removed.

12. 3. 4. 4   Statistical Models of Meta-Analysis

Several different formulae can be selected for combining results of a meta-analysis. The two most commonly used formulae are the "formula of fixed-effects model" and the "formula of random-effects model".

(1)Fixed-Effects Model

The fixed-effects model assumes that all included studies investigate the same population, use the same outcome definitions, and estimate the same intervention effect. It provides a weighted average of a series of study estimates. The inverse of the estimates' variance is commonly used as study weight, so that larger studies tend to contribute more than smaller studies to the weighted average. Consequently, when studies within a meta-analysis are dominated by a very large study, the findings from smaller studies are practically ignored. If all the studies had followed the same study protocol and were conducted at the same time (contemporaneously), the fixed-effects model could be used with little or no hesitation. Investigators often use this model for combining results across centers in multicentric studies.

(2)Random-Effects Model

The random-effects model assumes that the studies are not all estimating the same intervention effect but rather estimating intervention effects that follow a distribution across studies. This is the basis of a random-effects meta-analysis. The random-effects model is a common model used to synthesize heterogeneous research. This is simply the weighted average of the effect sizes of a group of studies. The weight applied in weighted averaging with a random effects meta-analysis is achieved in two steps: ①inverse variance weighting; ②unweighting of this inverse variance weighting by applying a random effects variance component (REVC) that is simply derived from the extent of variability of the effect sizes of the underlying studies.

The extent to which the protocol and timing of the studies differ will determine whether one model is justified over the other. The researcher may use both, and if both approaches yield the same conclusions, the conclusions are considered strong. If they differ, the conclusions are considered weak and more studies or other sources of evidence (e. g. , non-randomized studies) are necessary to support the conclusions.

12. 3. 5　General Approach to Pooling Data

12. 3. 5. 1　Types of Data

When we start pooling data in a meta-analysis, we should first identify the data type for the outcome measurements.

①Dichotomous (or binary) data: Each individual's outcome is one of only two possible categorical responses.

②Continuous data: Each individual's outcome is a measurement of a numerical quantity.

③Ordinal data (including measurement scales): The outcome is one of several ordered categories, or generated by scoring and summing categorical responses.

④Counts and rates.

⑤Time-to-event (typically survival) data.

12. 3. 5. 2　Effect Measures for Dichotomous Outcomes

The most common methods for measuring effects in clinical trials with dichotomous data are the risk ratio (RR, also called the relative risk), odds ratio (OR), risk difference (RD, also called the absolute risk reduction), and the number needed to treat (NNT) for an additional beneficial or harmful outcome.

12. 3. 5. 3　Effect Measures for Continuous Outcomes

The common effect measures used in clinical trials with continuous data are the mean difference (MD, or difference in means), which is a standard statistic that measures the ab-solute difference between the mean value in two groups in a clinical trial, standardized mean difference (SMD), and the weighted mean difference (WMD). MD and SMD are the two most commonly used summary statistics for meta-analysis of continuous data.

12. 3. 5. 4   Summarizing Effects Across Studies

The standard error of the pooled intervention effect of a meta-analysis can be used to derive a confidence interval (CI), which communicates the precision (or uncertainty) of the summary estimate, and to derive a P-value, which communicates the strength of the evi-dence against the null hypothesis of no intervention effect. $P \leqslant 0.05$ indicates that the pooled effect size of multiple studies is statistically significant. On the contrary, if $P > 0.05$, the pooled effect size is not statistically significant. Whenever the 95% CI crosses the line of null value (RR or OR=1 in dichotomous data or RD, MD or SMD=0 in continuous data) equate to $P > 0.05$. Several commonly used methods to summarize effects across studies are introduced below.

(1)A Generic Inverse-Variance Method

The inverse-variance method is a very common and simple version of the meta-analysis procedure and is used behind the scenes in certain meta-analyses of both dichotomous and continuous data. Through this approach, larger studies (which have smaller standard er-rors) are given more weight than smaller studies (which have larger standard errors). This choice of weight minimizes the imprecision (uncertainty) of the pooled effect estimate.

(2)Random-Effects (DerSimonian and Laird, D-L) Method

A random-effects method incorporates an assumption that different studies are estima-ting different, yet related, intervention effects. It's a variation from the inverse-variance method, and its simplest version is the D-L method.

(3)Mantel-Haenszel (M-H) Methods

M-H methods are the default fixed-effect methods in RevMan to conduct data pooling for a meta-analysis. When data are sparse, either in terms of event rates being low or study size being small, M-H methods use a different weighting scheme that depends upon which effect measure (e. g. , RR, OR, RD) is being used. M-H methods have been shown to have better statistical properties than inverse variance methods when there are few events.

(4)Peto Odds Ratio Method

Peto's method can only be used to pool OR. Peto's method is recommended when inter-vention effects are small (odds ratios are close to 1), events are not particularly common, and the studies have similar numbers in experimental and control groups. An alternative way of viewing the Peto method is as a sum of "O-E" statistics. Here, O is the observed number of events and E is an expected number of events in each study's experimental inter-vention group.

The summary of meta-analysis methods is shown in Table 12. 3.

Table 12.3   Summary of Meta-Analysis Methods

Type of Data	Effect Measure	Models*	Calculation Methods
Dichotomous	Odds ratio (OR)	Fixed-effect models	Peto
		Fixed-effect models	Mantel-Haenszel (M-H)
		Random-effects models	DerSimonian and Laird (D-L)
	Risk ratio (RR)	Fixed-effect models	Mantel-Haenszel (M-H)
		Random-effects models	DerSimonian and Laird (D-L)
	Risk difference (RD)	Fixed-effect models	Mantel-Haenszel (M-H)
		Random-effects models	DerSimonian and Laird (D-L)
Continuous	Mean difference (MD)	Fixed-effect models	inverse variance (IV)
		Random-effects models	DerSimonian and Laird (D-L)
	Standardized mean difference (SMD)	Fixed-effect models	inverse variance (IV)
		Random-effects models	DerSimonian and Laird (D-L)
O-E and variance	Odds ratio (OR)	Fixed-effect models	Peto

* After addressing heterogeneity, if $P \leqslant 0.1$ in a heterogeneity test, then use the random-effects model

12.3.5.5   Forest Plots

A forest plot shows effect estimates and confidence intervals for both individual studies and meta-analyses. Each study is represented by a block at the point where the intervention effect is estimated, with a horizontal line extending to both sides of the block. The block area represents the weight assigned to the study in the meta-analysis, while the horizontal line describes the confidence interval (usually 95% CI). The confidence interval describes the range of intervention effects consistent with the study results and indicates whether each intervention effect has a separate statistical significance. Wide blocks represent large weight studies (usually those with narrower confidence intervals) that dominate the calculation of the pooled results. The forest plot is a simple and intuitive way to represent meta-analysis statistical results, and it is the most commonly used form of result representation in meta-analyses.

An example of forest plots of using results from a review of compression stockings to prevent deep vein thrombosis (DVT) in airline passengers is given in Figure 12.1.

12.3.6   Addressing Reporting Biases

12.3.6.1   What Are Reporting Biases?

The dissemination of research findings is not a division into published or unpublished, but a continuum ranging from the sharing of draft papers among colleagues, through presentations at meetings and published abstracts, to papers in journals that are indexed in the major bibliographic databases. It has long been recognized that only a proportion of research

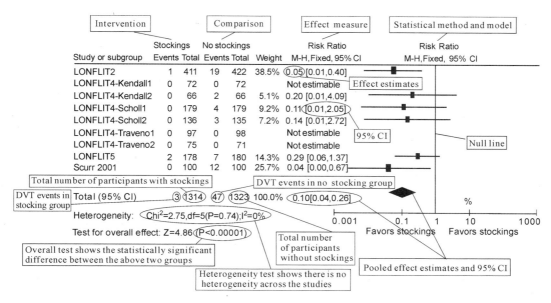

Figure 12. 1   Example of Forest Plots

projects ultimately reach publication in an indexed journal and thus become easily identifiable for meta-analyses or systematic reviews. Reporting biases arise when the dissemination of research findings is influenced by the nature and direction of results. This means the "positive" results indicating that intervention works are more likely to be published, published rapidly, published in English, published more than once, published in high-impact journals and, more likely to be cited by others. One important note: the contribution made to the totality of the evidence by studies with non-significant results is as important as that from studies with statistically significant results.

12. 3. 6. 2   Types of Reporting Biases

Various types of reporting bias exist, including publication bias, time-lag bias, duplicate publication bias. Some types of reporting biases and their definitions are listed in Table 12. 4.

Table 12. 4   Definitions of Some Types of Reporting Biases

Type of Reporting Bias	Definition
Publication bias	The publication or non-publication of research findings, depending on the nature and direction of the results
Time-lag bias	The rapid or delayed publication of research findings, depending on the nature and direction of the results
Multiple (duplicate) publication bias	The multiple or singular publication of research findings, depending on the nature and direction of the results
Location bias	The publication of research findings in journals with different ease of access or levels of indexing in standard databases, depending on the nature and direction of results

(To be continued)

Table 12. 4

Type of Reporting Bias	Definition
Citation bias	The citation or non-citation of research findings, depending on the nature and direction of the results
Language bias	The publication of research findings in a particular language, depending on the nature and direction of the results
Outcome-reporting bias	The selective reporting of some outcomes but not others, depending on the nature and direction of the results
Database bias	The publication of research findings in databases with different levels of indexing, depending on the nature and direction of results
Inclusion bias	The inclusion or exclusion of research findings according to a specified inclusion criterion for a meta-analysis, depending on the nature and direction of the results
Selector bias	The selection or non-selection of research findings, depending on the nature and direction of the results

12. 3. 6. 3　Detecting Reporting Biases

(1) Funnel Plots

The "funnel plot" is so named because the precision of the estimated intervention effect increases as the size of the study increases. A funnel plot is a simple scatter plot of the intervention effect estimates from individual studies against some measures of each study's size or precision. It is most common to plot the effect estimates on the horizontal scale and the measure of study size on the vertical axis (Figure 12. 2). Effect estimates from small studies will, therefore, scatter more widely at the bottom of the graph, with the spread narrowing among larger studies. In the absence of bias, the plot should approximately resemble a symmetrical (inverted) funnel. If there is bias, for example, because smaller studies without statistically significant effects (shown as open circles in Figure 12. 2 remain unpublished, this will lead to an asymmetrical appearance of the funnel plot with a gap in a bottom corner of the graph (Figure 12. 3). In this situation, the effect calculated in a meta-analysis will

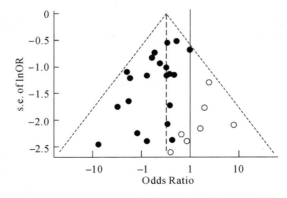

Figure 12. 2　Symmetrical Plot in the Absence of Bias

tend to overestimate the intervention effect. The more pronounced the asymmetry, the more likely the amount of bias will be substantial. But an asymmetrical funnel plot should not be equated with publication bias; differences in methodological quality are an important source of the asymmetry funnel plot.

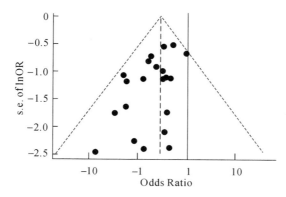

Figure 12. 3   Asymmetrical Plot in the Presence of Bias

(2) Sensitivity Analysis

When authors find evidence of small-study effects, they should consider sensitivity analyses to examine how the results of the meta-analysis change under different assumptions relating to the reasons for these effects.

(3) Fail-Safe N

Fail-safe N is the number of research studies required to overthrow or reverse the current combined results. The greater the fail-safe N, the more stable the meta-analysis results, and the less likely the results are to be overthrown. This method is easy to conduct. The disadvantage is that it cannot be applied when the combined effect size is not statistically significant.

Although there is clear evidence that publication and other reporting biases lead to over-optimistic estimates of intervention effects, overcoming, detecting and correcting for publication bias is problematic. Comprehensive searching is important to prevent publication bias, but comprehensive searching alone is not sufficient to prevent some substantial potential biases. Publication bias should be regarded as one of the possible causes of small-study effects. Funnel plots allow researchers to make a visual assessment of whether small-study effects are present in a meta-analysis, and the results from tests for funnel plot asymmetry should be interpreted cautiously.

12.3.6.4   Strategies for Avoiding Reporting Biases

Several measures can be taken to reduce or avoid reporting biases.

①Undertake a comprehensive search for studies that meet the eligibility criteria for a meta-analysis. Authors should ensure they search multiple sources. For example, the Cochrane Central Register of Controlled Trials (CENTRAL), MEDLINE, and EMBASE should all be searched for a qualified meta-analysis.

②Include unpublished studies. Obtaining and including data from unpublished trials appears to be one obvious way of avoiding publication bias.

③Enroll in prospective trial registration, which has the potential to reduce the effects of publication bias substantially.

④Implement objective and rigorous inclusion criteria and blind screening. These are the most important methods to control the selector's biases.

⑤Interpret results objectively.

A meta-analysis combines the intervention effect estimates across included studies. Since it is possible that studies suggesting a beneficial intervention effect or a larger effect size are published, while a similar amount of data that points in the other direction remain unpublished, a meta-analysis of the published studies could potentially identify a spurious beneficial intervention effect or miss an important adverse intervention effect. Therefore, when we plan to conclude the meta-analysis, we should consider the following two points: ①Is there enough evidence and is it strong enough to suggest an intervention is "effective" or "ineffective"? ②Do the results of the meta-analysis indicate a direction for further research? If so, continue the research and update the analysis.

12.3.7 Advantages and Disadvantages of Meta-Analysis

12.3.7.1 Advantages of Meta-Analysis

The main advantage of meta-analysis is an increase in power. Power is the chance of detecting a real effect as statistically significant, if it exists. Many individual studies are too small to detect small effects but when several are combined, there is a higher chance of detecting the weak effect.

Meta-analyses can also improve precision. The estimation of an intervention effect can be improved when it is based on more information, which means that the combined result may be more precise and, hence, often conclusive, even when individual studies are inconclusive. Conclusive results of a meta-analysis on a topic may obviate the need for a new trial and expedite the application of the research results. Even when results are inconclusive, meta-analysis defines the area for research, generates hypotheses to be tested and informs future research regarding limitations of the available evidence. Experts believe that the results of meta-analysis have greater generalizability because they are based on a variety of study populations. For a given topic, the summary provided by a meta-analysis is useful for economic evaluation, decision analysis, and clinical practice guidelines.

A meta-analysis can answer questions not posed by individual studies. Primary studies often involve a specific type of patient and explicitly defined interventions. A selection of studies in which these characteristics differ can allow investigation of the effect's consistency and, if relevant, allow investigation into the reasons for differences in effect estimates.

Another advantage of meta-analysis is its utility in settling controversies that arise from apparently conflicting studies or in generating new hypotheses. Statistical analysis of findings allows the degree of conflict to be formally assessed, and reasons for different results to be explored and quantified.

12.3.7.2　Disadvantages of Meta-Analysis

Meta-Analyses also have the potential to mislead seriously, particularly if specific study designs, within-study biases, variation across studies, and reporting biases are not carefully considered.

All meta-analyses must deal with publication bias; that is, positive results are published more often than negative ones. Thus, a meta-analysis based on only published trials may yield a false-positive result. Such instances have already occurred in the medical literature. Another limitation is its infeasibility when the studies have used different outcomes or have measured outcomes differently or the reports do not include some vital aspect of the study and authors are unavailable or apathetic. A problem often called "combining apples and oranges" refers to combining very dissimilar studies, which may drown a genuine positive result into an overall false negative conclusion.

12.4　Reporting Guidelines of Systematic Review

12.4.1　Introduction to PRISMA

PRISMA (Preferred Reporting Items of Systematic Reviews and Meta-Analyses) is an evidence-based minimum set of items for reporting systematic reviews and meta-analyses. PRISMA focuses on the reporting of reviews evaluating randomized trials, but it can also be used as a basis for reporting systematic reviews of other types of research, particularly evaluations of interventions. A PRISMA statement consists of a 27-item checklist and a four-stage flow diagram. The checklist contains the necessary items for a transparent systematic review. The PRISMA statement is designed to help authors improve the reporting of systematic reviews and meta-analyses, and it may also be useful for critical appraisal of published systematic reviews. However, the PRISMA checklist is not a quality assessment instrument and is not intended to gauge the quality of a systematic review.

12.4.2　PRISMA Flow Diagram

The flow diagram depicts the flow of information through the different phases of a systematic review. It maps out the number of records identified, included and excluded, and the reasons for exclusions (Figure 12.4). The PRISMA flow diagram has been modified based on the QUOROM flow diagram. Before including studies and providing reasons for excluding others, the review team must record the retrieval results in detail. The PRISMA flow diagram now requests information on these phases of the review process to capture this information.

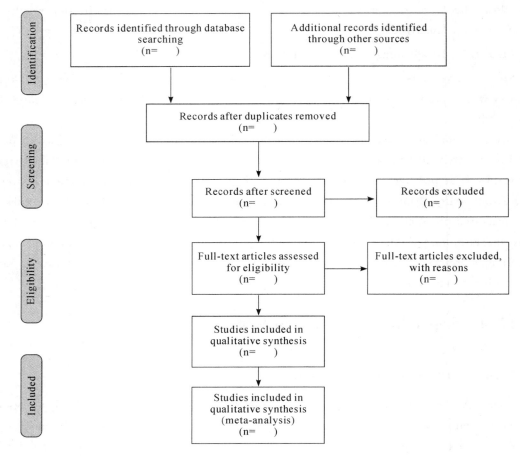

Figure 12. 4   PRISMA Flow Diagram

12. 4. 3   PRISMA Checklist

The 27 checklist items pertain to the content of a systematic review and meta-analysis, which include the title, the abstract, methods, results, discussions, and funding (http://www. prisma-statement. org/). The new PRISMA checklist differs in several respects from the QUOROM checklist. It "decouples" several items present in the QUOROM checklist and, where applicable, several checklist items are linked to improving consistency across the systematic review report.

(Tang Shaowen, Jing Yuanyuan, Wang Hui, Zhao Jinshun)

Exercise

Chapter 13   Interpretation of Epidemiologic Literature

13. 1   Introduction

A 40-year-old taxi driver visited his family physician for an annual checkup. The patient's father had been diagnosed with colorectal cancer in the past year, and the patient wanted advice about what he could do to reduce his own risk of developing this cancer. In responding to the patient's questions about colorectal cancer, the physician confirmed that a positive family history augments the risk of developing this disease. A certain number of other behaviors are associated with a reduced risk of developing colorectal cancer, such as consumption of abundant fresh vegetables and fruits, but the factors predisposing a patient to develop a disease are not easy to modify. The physician was aware of the controversy regarding dietary fat intake and the occurrence of cancer. Before providing a recommendation about fat intake, the physician wished to review the pertinent medical literature.

The recommendations that physicians give to patients depend on the current state of available knowledge about diseases, the underlying pathophysiology of diseases, and the most effective treatment for diseases. The knowledge base of clinical medicine is constantly expanding, and physicians must, therefore, develop methods to uncover and apply new information. This process is complicated when inconclusive or conflicting results are found in the literature. The publication of articles, even in the most reputable journals, cannot guarantee that the investigator's conclusions are valid and practical. The history of medicine includes examples of therapies that were once generally accepted but were later proved to be ineffective or even harmful to patients. Clinicians should always stay abreast of new knowledge and keep developing skills that enable them to provide the appropriate care to the patients.

13. 2   Literature Searches

The first step in updating medical knowledge is to seek the proper documents, which is an increasingly difficult assignment. No physician can read all the related literature immediately, especially since the number of publications increases each year. Luckily, with the help of various tools, literature searches can be achieved easily. Generally, the medical literature searching process can be divided into four parts: ①framing pertinent clinical questions; ②selecting a literature database; ③making a search strategy; and ④choosing appropriate literature.

The most popular online resource to start searching for medical papers is PubMed (https://www.ncbi.nlm.nih.gov/pubmed/), a free search engine owned by the National Library of Medicine, which also provides access to MEDLINE, PreMEDLINE, and the Cochrane Database of Systematic Reviews. Additionally, general search engines, such as Google Scholar and Baidu, have been broadly applied to provide access to free published articles. Since these databases do not overlap totally, it is worth searching all to confirm comprehensive coverage. The searching methods of different search engines might vary; however, the fundamental principles are applied across the board. For simplicity, this chapter will concentrate on the PubMed database.

The search strategy is based on the main research concepts, which means the study hypothesis should determine the terms used to search the literature. In addition, the search should be reproducible. An experienced medical librarian can be invaluable in designing and implementing a comprehensive search. The search terms should be cross-checked with the experts to ensure that the proper studies are detected and that any systematic bias related to the search strategy is avoided.

The Medical Subject Headings (MeSH) is a comprehensive thesaurus of key words developed by the National Library of Medicine of the United States to cover all topics in biomedicine. The MeSH browser (http://www.nlm.nih.gov/mesh/meshhome.html) can automatically branch out to search for related or alternate terms and spellings so that one does not need to identify and search those respectively. Based on the specific MeSH term used, this feature can cast a very broad net. Nonetheless, at this point of search, one would like to be precise, and it is easy to remove non-relevant studies or missing literature by too-narrow searches. The MeSH browser should be applied to identify the relevant MeSH terms for the study question.

MeSH terms do have one limitation. Because the process of indexing articles and using the relevant MeSH terms and features to filter the search results is time-consuming, the MeSH browser is not always up to date; that is, recently published articles presented in PubMed may not be collected by a search that relies entirely on MeSH terms. If one is researching a topic that has been receiving an extensive amount of recent attention, one might need to add free text-terms as well as MeSH terms to avoid missing the most recent documents.

Once search terms are determined, PubMed permits search terms to be combined using Boolean connectors (e.g., AND, OR, NOT). Beginners could acquire more information from the online tutorial (http://www.nlm.nih.gov/bsd/disted/pubmedtutorial/cover.html). In the example of dietary fat intake and the risk of developing colorectal cancer, a search like the following might be used: "dietary fats" [MeSH Terms] AND "colorectal neoplasms" [MeSH Terms] AND "risk". This search generates far more results than the relevant literature that will answer our questions. For example, it will gather editorials which are not original research results. PubMed provides tools that can filter our unwanted articles; for instance, the search results might be restricted to ①article types—cohort studies, case-control studies, systematic reviews or meta-analyses; ② species—humans; ③ language—English; and ④publication period, which could reduce the number of articles to an acceptable amount.

13.3   Reviewing Individual Studies

Once the appropriate articles are selected, it is useful to apply a uniform and comprehensive approach to assess the literature. This procedure urges readers to consider all aspects of a study before making an opinion on its validity and utility. The following paragraphs provide such a procedure for evaluating individual published papers (Table 13.1). Each step is somewhat dependent on other steps, and they are often considered to be integrated. The reader should consider internal validity, external validity, and clinical practice as crucial factors in assessing collected studies.

Table 13.1   Procedure for Evaluating Individual Published Papers

Internal Validity

Step 1. Consider the research hypothesis.

Does the study have a clear research hypothesis?

Does the study question have clinical relevance?

Step 2. Consider the study design.

Does the study use experimental or observational methods?

Can the study design fulfil the hypothesis?

Is the design better than previous approaches?

Step 3. Consider the outcome variable.

Is the outcome related to clinical practice?

What's the definition of the disease of interest?

Is the determination of the occurrence or absence of disease precise?

Step 4. Consider the predictor variables.

How many exposures or risk factors are being studied?

What's the definition of exposure?

Is the measurement of exposure accurate?

Will the duration of exposure be quantified?

Are biological markers of exposure used in the research?

(To be continued)

Table 13. 1

Step 5. Consider the method of analysis.

Are the applied statistical methods proper for the types of variables in the study? (category or continuous one?)

Have the levels of type I and type Ⅱ errors been discussed appropriately?

Is the sample size adequate to answer the research question?

Did the statistical tests meet the underlying assumption?

Has opportunity been evaluated as a potential explanation of the results?

Step 6. Consider the possible sources of bias.

Is there any selection bias?

Is there any information bias?

Is there any confounding bias?

In what direction would each potential bias influence the results?

External Validity

Step 7. Consider how the results of the study can be extrapolated to the general population.

Are results consistent with other studies according to the same question?

Can the findings be applied to other human population?

Do the findings suggest a change in current clinical practice?

Clinical Practice

Step 8. Consider how the results of the study can be used in practice.

How large is the observed effect?

Is there a dose-response relationship?

Are the findings in line with laboratory models?

Are the effects biologically plausible?

If the findings are negative, was there sufficient statistical power to detect an effect?

Adapted from Shen Hongbing, Zheng Zhijie, Zhao Yashuang, et al. *Epidemiology*. Beijing: People Medicine Publishing House, 2018

13. 3. 1　Research Hypothesis

It is important to identify the study's research hypothesis. This can be difficult since authors often are not straightforward in stating their hypothesis. Sometimes the goal of the study is declared as a study question and sometimes the reader can only identify the goal of the study by understanding a set of complicated analyses.

Once the aim of the study is discerned, the reader should distinguish whether the study has clinical importance. If the study does not, the finding may have little relevance to clinical practice.

For the physician who requires information to answer a patient about the association between dietary fat and colorectal cancer, it is necessary to identify the literature that addresses this topic. For instance, research on the effects of varying dietary fat composition on the occurrence of colorectal tumors in mice may be useful, because studies carried out in laboratory animals can be tightly controlled for those confounding factors. However, it may be more useful to read a study on the effect of a high-fat diet on circulating carcinogenic factors to the large intestine. Since this study may be relevant to the biological plausibility of a potential relationship between dietary fat and colorectal cancer. This type of research may reveal the underlying mechanism of disease development and prevention.

The reader also should distinguish various types of significance ascribed by research. It is common to base the significance of a study's results on statistical evidence. The evaluation of statistical significance refers to the likelihood of committing a type I error as well, which can help the reader to interpret results. However, even if a finding is statistically significant, it may not be clinically or biologically significant. For example, a small difference in the risk of developing colorectal cancer with an elevated amount of dietary fat could be statistically significant if the finding was based on a huge number of observations. Nonetheless, the risk of this evaluation may be so tiny that an individual's risk of developing colorectal cancer would not be appreciably altered by changing his/her dietary pattern. As a result, a clinical recommendation to reduce dietary fat by changing his/her diet might not be supported. The biological significance of a finding reveals another issue: do the epidemiological observations help to clarify the causal mechanism? Those types of results are most likely to be gained if the epidemiological studies are performed to test the association between biological markers of exposure, susceptibility, and outcomes.

13.3.2 Study Design

Once a reader finds a research aim of interest, he/she should determine what kind of study design was implemented. Certain type of designs may be useful in answering specific kinds of questions. Additionally, the investigators' current state of knowledge will impact their choice of study design. Previous studies on a hypothesis may have a simple design (e. g. , descriptive study). As the hypothesis is refined, a more rigorous study design should be applied.

The suitability of the research design for the study question should be evaluated. The incidence rate of the disease of interest might be a determining factor. For instance, although colorectal cancer is the most common cancer among the whole population, the disease is diagnosed among only a small percentage of people within a short period. Thus, a case-control study would be chosen as an efficient approach to investigate the cause of this disease, since the participants were enrolled once they were diagnosed. In practice, studies on dietary fat intake and the occurrence of colorectal cancer have implemented several different designs, including descriptive, case-control, cohort studies, and clinical trials. Descriptive studies are useful for hypothesis generation, but not for hypothesis testing. Cohort studies and case-control studies provide stronger evidence to test certain hypotheses. Randomized controlled trials are the optimal solution for verifying a hypothesis.

13. 3. 3　Outcome Variables

The outcome of interest in the patient profile is the development of colorectal cancer. In searching for the association between dietary fat consumption and the risk of colorectal cancer, the reader should define the occurrence and absence of colorectal cancer. Several possibilities exist.

①Death certificates restrict the information to deceased subjects. Also, a variety of studies have shown that the information on death certificates may not be accurate.

②Self-reports require subjects to be alive or have friends or relatives who can provide information about their colorectal cancer. If the subjects are not familiar with medical terms, they might misunderstand benign forms of the colorectal disease for colorectal cancer.

③Medical records may provide more precise information than death certificates or self-reports. However, the diagnostic criteria may differ from hospital to hospital, from time to time or between countries.

④Histopathologic diagnoses provide the most definitive information, but appropriate tissue must be available for pathologic examinations.

It is desirable to have the most accurate information possible about the disease of interest. This minimizes the possibility of the misclassification of subjects. For colorectal cancer, a small proportion of apparently healthy people may have occult colorectal cancer. This could be verified by a screening test, such as biomarker testing (Cancer Embryo Antigen, CEA), or colonoscopy, on all apparently unaffected subjects. Since so few asymptomatic cancers are likely to be detected, however, the study findings would probably not be greatly affected by limiting the detection to routine histopathologic diagnosis.

Judging the accuracy of an investigator's outcomes is critical. In general, a practical approach is to specify a single simple disease entity when searching for causes. For instance, a study of dietary fat and the risk of all cancers combined may provide misleading results, since different cancers have different risk factors and only a few may involve dietary fat. Limiting the study to colorectal cancer improves the likelihood of acquiring a confirmed result for this disease of interest.

13. 3. 4　Predictor Variables

The predictor variable is the risk factor or exposure under investigation. A single risk factor or various risk factors of interest may be involved in one study. If several exposure variables are included, they may or may not be closely correlated.

In a study on the cause of colorectal cancer, a researcher may want to investigate a variety of exposure variables, including family history, age, sex, physical activity and dietary fat intake. Although this kind of study can provide a more comprehensive picture of the causes of colorectal cancer, it may be restricted by the ability to collect all the information on each risk factor of interest. Even if a study is focused on the association between dietary fat and colorectal cancer, the researcher must collect basic information on the possible colorectal cancer determinants that may act as confounders.

The reader should distinguish whether the methods applied to characterize the occurrence and absence of risk factors are reliable and accurate. Possible methods of confirmation include subject or surrogate respondent reports, direct observation, or measurement of a biological marker. The reader should ask whether better ways are available to define subjects' exposure levels.

Even the evaluation of dietary exposure could be difficult. In one approach, subjects are asked to recall what they regularly eat, using a common food frequency questionnaire. Various studies have revealed that this kind of recall, although imperfect, may be adequate to determine whether a subject consumes a relatively high, moderate, or low amount of dietary fat. Generally, acquiring several levels of exposures is desirable, and thus a dose-response relationship can be measured as well.

Another approach to determining dietary fat intake is to ask subjects to record what they currently eat. This can be achieved by writing a diary or by checking a list of commonly eaten foods to select the meals and snacks being consumed. This approach has limitations as well. For instance, subjects may forget to record what they have eaten or the proportion, which is very hard to estimate precisely, and may not be accurate. To offset such problems, plastic models of different portion sizes may be provided to subjects for quantification. Of note, a subject's current diet may not accurately reflect his/her past diet pattern. In a case-control study mostly based on the current diet information, it is critical to know if subjects with colorectal cancer changed their diets because of the disease, the side effects of treatment, or the hope of influencing prognosis.

The third approach to collecting diet information is to measure what subjects eat. This could be practical for a prospective cohort study in which subjects are followed to identify whether they develop colorectal cancer in the future. Indeed, this approach would be extremely difficult to implement, since it requires a strictly controlled environment in which the researcher could record all the foods the subjects eat.

Sometimes, epidemiologists use the advantage of a situation in which people maintain a certain dietary pattern for religious or other reasons. For example, vegetarians consume very little fat. The occurrence of colorectal cancer in this group of people could be compared with another group of people who consume a large amount of fat. However, the accuracy of measuring the amount of fat consumed in a diet is still a problem. Furthermore, other confounders, such as lifestyle factors in both groups may also influence the development of colorectal cancer.

Currently, using biological markers of exposure is becoming more common in clinical research. Biological markers are crucial because they can be quantified. No biological markers of diet fat are available yet, but to assess long-term intake of dietary fat, the fatty acid content of adipose tissue could be measured in biopsies. Obviously, the implementation of such a measure relies on the extent to which it accurately reflects consumption patterns. The willingness of study subjects to agree with a tissue biopsy must also be considered.

13.3.5　Methods of Analysis

At the core of a research finding is the ability to exclude chance as an explanation for the results. This could be achieved by statistical tests. Readers should have a basic knowledge of which statistical tests are suitable for which kind of data. The type of statistical test that should be used is determined by the aim of the analysis and the types of variables used in the analysis.

Generally, the α is set at a level of 5% statistical significance in most biomedical studies. Thus, the researcher would like to agree a 1 in 20 risk that the observed effect is the result of chance alone. However, the author should be careful when explaining the meaning of P-value. One common mistake is to assume that a statistical significance is equal to biological or clinical importance. As mentioned above, clinical and biological importance is not assessed by the statistical tests.

A second common mistake is to ignore a finding since it has not achieved the pre-established level of statistical significance. A P-value of 0.08, for instance, it is not statistically significant by convention. However, it still represents a result that is relatively unlikely to be caused by chance. It would be unconscionable to conclude only based on the P-value that no association was detected between dietary fat and colorectal cancer in a study. A strong reliance on the P-value is dangerous when the sample size is relatively small and the statistical power is low as well. In such circumstance, even moderate differences between groups may not reach the pre-established statistical significance, which means the possibility of reaching a solid conclusion is limited.

13.3.6　Possible Sources of Bias

A finding must be evaluated to distinguish whether it could be caused by systematic errors introduced by selecting samples or data collection procedures. The statistical method cannot indicate what kinds of biases are responsible for the detected results. Bias can occur in any research, although certain designs are more prone to specific types of bias. Three major biases should be considered in most research regardless of the study design.

The first concern is whether the selected sample can represent the target population. Since few new kinds of research can test the whole population, the investigator will usually select a certain sample to make inferences about the whole population. The reader should determine whether the samples represent the population and what extrapolation is made.

The methods described in any published medical literature should include detailed information about how the participants are chosen. In a case-control study, typical selection bias would arise from the approach used to select patients and controls from a certain hospital. In the context of a case-control study on dietary fat and colorectal cancer, a selection bias might occur if prevalent cases are used rather than newly diagnosed cases. For example, if a person consumed a high-fat diet before developing colorectal cancer, but reduced his/her consumption of fat after being diagnosed with colorectal cancer, this person may report the current, reduced-fat diet to the interviewer and this will appear as the reason for the subject's survival.

In a case-control study, the sampling of controls would be the most difficult aspect and also the most susceptible to selection bias. Consider a hospital-based sample of control subjects with the diagnosis of other diseases rather than colorectal cancer. If the disease of the control participants is caused by dietary factors, e. g. , breast cancer, or if the disease impacts dietary intake, e. g. , gastritis, then a biased case-control comparison may ensue. Sampling controls from the general population would better reflect the exposure pattern of persons without the disease of interest. However, even the general population sampling method could introduce bias. For instance, a telephone sampling technique might preferentially enroll higher-income members, because they are more likely to have a telephone in their home compared with lower-income members. Furthermore, higher-income members are less likely to work outside; therefore, they would be more often chosen when the sampling is conducted. Because the diet of the higher-income population may differ from that of the lower-income population, a biased control comparison may occur. To explore whether a telephone sampling procedure will yield an unbiased sample of control subjects, the researcher should identify the coverage of the telephone in the target population. Furthermore, multiple calls should be performed at different periods to ensure that people who work outside the home can be reached.

Cohort studies are prone to a potential selection bias as well. The most notable selection bias is the loss to follow-up. If persons who usually had a high-fat diet tend to migrate or discontinue participation in the cohort study for other reasons before the diagnosis of cancer, the investigator will underestimate the association between dietary fat consumption and colorectal cancer. Currently, the bias of loss to follow-up in cohort studies has generated controversial results. When evaluating cohort studies, the reader should consider to what extent the bias would occur due to loss to follow-up.

Another major bias is named information bias or misclassification bias. For instance, in a case-control study, exposure status is normally collected after diagnosis with a disease of interest. Mostly, subjects are aware of their disease and have undergone related treatment, and their reporting of past exposures may systematically differ from the reporting of controls. This is also called recall bias. Studies on dietary risk factors are susceptible to recall bias. For instance, if patients with colorectal cancer notice the association between dietary fat and colorectal cancer, they might overestimate past intake of dietary fat. Controls may be less concerned about their past diet or may be less worried about their diet, which would tend to make them underreport their exposure status.

If recall bias existed in a study, the investigator might overestimate the association between dietary fat intake and the risk of developing colorectal cancer. In fact, abundant of studies have illustrated problems of imprecise recall in dietary information collection. Only a few studies have compared the differential recall in cases versus controls by retrospectively collecting dietary data with subsequent data that was prospectively collected from the same subjects. Overall, research has not illustrated a differential recall of food intake in the cases of colorectal cancer in comparison with controls. This might indicate that recall bias is an unlikely explanation for those conflicting results that are detected from case-control studies on the relationship between dietary fat intake and colorectal cancer.

It should be noted, even if cases and controls have the same ability to recall dietary exposure, misclassification bias could still happen. Errors in reporting that are comparable between the cases and controls would introduce non-differential misclassification. If non-differential misclassification occurs, it may decrease the estimated odds ratio. In other words, such misclassification tends to make it more difficult to find any true differences between cases and controls.

Another important consideration of bias is to discern the confounding bias. A confounder is the third variable that correlates with both the disease of interest and the risk factor being examined. It accounts for some or all of the observed associations between the risk factor and the disease. In research on the relationship between dietary fat intake and the development of colorectal cancer, the reader must check whether the investigator accounted for the effects of known risk factors for colorectal cancer. These factors include age, race, family history, smoking, drinking, and physical activity. If the person who consumed a high-fat diet was less physically active than those who eat a low-fat diet, an apparent association between consumption of fat and the occurrence of colorectal cancer could be attributed to the effects of physical activity rather than the effects of diet.

In an observational study, confounders could be controlled either by matching the subject with known confounders or by restricting the subject's inclusion criteria during the study design step. Confounders could even be processed by statistical analysis after data collection. All these adjustment methods are based on the variables known to be confounders. For other unknown risk factors, matching or adjustment plays a limited role. Any observed association between dietary fat intake and the occurrence of colorectal cancer could be explained partially in that way.

If a potential bias exists, estimating both the magnitude and the direction of the bias is worthwhile, because these factors could impact the result. In this way, the reader can distinguish if the bias is likely to overestimate or underestimate the effect of exposure. In a case-control study, for instance, if it is suspected that people with colorectal cancer are more likely to remember and report fat intake compared with controls, the odds ratio could be overestimated. In contrast, if it seems that persons with colorectal cancer are likely to under-report their fat intake compared with their controls, the odds ratio could be underestimated. In discussing the results, an investigator may attempt to convince the reader that the magnitude of bias would not be sufficient to skew the results, or that the true relationship is stronger than what was observed.

13. 3. 7 Interpretation of Results

If, after reviewing results from the literature, the reader finds the statistical significance cannot be attributed to biases, then the reader should consider whether the result is clinically important. For instance, one study revealed a 50% decrease in dietary fat intake related to a 5% reduction in risk of developing colorectal cancer. Although the result is statistically significant, the magnitude of the reduction in risk is small and individual patients may be poorly motivated to make the dietary change. However, the societal benefit of reducing 5% of all colorectal cancer cases may well justify a mass public education effort to decrease consumption of dietary fat. Thus, various types of significance should be distinguished during the study (Table 13. 2).

Table 13. 2 Interpretation Significance of Results

Type	Meaning	Assessment
Statistical	Exclusion of chance as an explanation for findings	Statistical test
Clinical	Importance of findings for changing current clinical practice	Magnitude of clinical response to an intervention
Biological	Usefulness of findings to clarify the mechanism of action	Comparison of findings to information from in vitro and in vivo laboratory experiments

Adapted from Shen Hongbing, Zheng Zhijie, Zhao Yashuang, et al. *Epidemiology*. Beijing: People Medicine Publishing House, 2018

13. 3. 8 Practical Utility of Results

When reviewing published research, the reader should consider the practical utility of the results. The usefulness of a study result depends on multiple factors, including the aim of the study, the representativeness of the subjects, and the consistency with finding from other published literature. Epidemiological and clinical studies have various purposes. The clinical utility of a certain research finding must be viewed in the context of the type of question raised. A study may direct to results related to disease causation, early detection of disease, the prediction of prognosis, or improved treatment. Unfortunately, no standard criteria exist to judge whether an association between a risk factor and a disease is clinically important. Normally, the stronger the association (i. e. , the risk ratio is far from the null value), the greater the potential benefit of eliminating the exposure. When evaluating clinical utility, one should consider the difficulty of changing the risk factor and the rate of morbidity and mortality associated with the disease of interest.

The ability to extrapolate findings from the literature to the general population should be considered as well. For instance, some studies on the risk factors of colorectal cancer are focused on the Caucasian population. This may limit the ability of such studies to be extrapolated to the Asian or African population. Researchers are mostly forced to restrict the sample by age, sex, race, or other factors. Readers must then determine whether these restrictions would affect the study's application to his/her own aim. To achieve this purpose, it is useful to evaluate whether other studies have obtained similar findings. Often, the first assessment of a potential risk factor, diagnostic test, or therapeutic regimen is favorable, while subsequent studies illustrate more limited applications. One possible reason for this situation is that initial evaluations often involve purposely selected subjects that represent a best-case scenario. Consequently, the following research tries to enlarge the application scope, which may prove to be less successful.

13. 4　Establishing a Causal Relationship

Finally, the reader may ask whether a study's finding proves a causal relationship between the risk factor and the development of a disease. Determining whether a causal relationship exists requires an examination of a certain study's results within the context of what is documented in the literature.

The temporal relationship between a suspected cause and an effect is vital; in other words, a cause must always precede an effect in time. This seems reasonable, but, in reality, factors suspected to be causes sometimes turn out to be consequences of a disease. For instance, a person with early undiagnosed cancer may change food preference due to some unknown systematic change of cancer. Therefore, the dietary change may be regarded as the cause of later diagnosed cancer. Case-control studies of chronic diseases with long latent periods are easily susceptible to this kind of problem. For a factor to be regarded as the cause of a disease, it is theoretically important to remove or modify that factor to decrease the incidence rate or mortality rate of the disease. However, in practice, eliminating or modifying a suspected causal factor may not always be possible. There are some examples in which a causal factor may trigger a protracted chain of events. Once set up, the sequence may no longer depend on the appearance of the causal agent for development. For instance, many cancers are thought to progress in response to an initiating event, followed by promotional effects that occur for many years. If the risk factor of interest only imitates the carcinogenesis, removal of the exposure during the promotional phase will not affect the subsequent risk of developing cancer. Therefore, the removal of an initiating risk factor for cancer may not affect the incidence of this disease for many years in the future.

Another criterion would be the strength of the association between risk factors and the disease. Usually, the strength of association is indicated by the risk ratio or odds ratio. When both values are far from the null value, the association is very strong, implying that the association is unlikely to be caused by chance or bias. Weak associations might also be causal, indicating only a slight risk of developing the disease. Caution should be paid to weak association, which might be caused by bias or chance.

It is useful to detect whether a dose-response relationship exists between a suspected risk factor and the disease, because increased levels of risk factor will be associated with a greater risk of developing the disease (or with protection in the case of protective factor). For instance, as the level of dietary fat intake increases, one would expect the risk of developing colorectal cancer to be elevated if there is a causal relationship. However, the absence of a progressive, graded dose-response relationship does not exclude a causal relationship. There may be a threshold of the risk conferring to the disease. In this example, the risk of disease will not be affected by the alternation of exposure concentration under a certain level, but the risk varies with a higher exposure level.

With any association, it is helpful to compare the findings with the results of other research. If other studies that use different populations under different settings get similar results, a causal relationship is confirmed. However, the reader must be careful when determining the consistency of those results, since it is possible that the same limitations could lead to an incorrect conclusion in several studies.

The supposed causal relationship should be in line with what is currently known about the biology and the disease process. This is often termed biological plausibility. If the proposed cause-and-effect relationship is not consistent with current biological knowledge, the causality may be doubted. The assessment of biological plausibility often requires a review of research on other human populations, as well as a review of studies that apply laboratory animal models.

13. 5 Summary

This chapter presented a structured procedure to interpret published epidemiological studies. The final goal of this approach is to translate epidemiological evidence into clinical practice. As a point for discussion, the instance of dietary fat intake and the risk of colorectal cancer was adopted to illustrate the interpreting process.

The first step in reviewing medical studies is to perform a thorough search for relevant publications. Selecting appropriate documents can be achieved through a manual or computer-assisted approach. In either situation, the correct selection of search terms is critical to extract relevant articles. Because they can save time, computer searches are preferred and popular.

Reviewing a publication starts with identifying the purpose of the research. For medical subjects, a primary consideration is whether this study demonstrates a clinically important question. Would the findings influence patient treatment strategies? In the present context, the clinical importance might be assessed in terms of whether the results support a suggestion to reduce dietary fat intake to decrease the risk of developing colorectal cancer.

The design of a study determines the types of causal inferences that can be concluded from it. The most solid evidence of a cause-effect relationship is derived from randomized controlled clinical trials. Among observational studies, prospective cohort studies generally present the strongest evidence, followed by retrospective cohort studies and case-control studies. Descriptive studies are useful for generating a research hypothesis but not for hypothesis testing. The measurement of exposure and outcome could be very difficult and complicated in observational studies. As much as possible, the investigator should try to acquire the most accurate information. In addition, assessments should be conducted in a blinded way and should be based on objective and standard criteria whenever possible.

A distinction must be made between the concept of statistical significance, which can be assessed by a hypothesis test, and of biological and clinical significance. P-values should not be used to imply the importance of a result, but rather, the possibility that sampling variability can explain the findings. Biological significance indicates the extent to which a finding helps to illustrate the underlying biological mechanism. Clinical utility relates to the difference in outcomes detected between the study groups and if these differences are large enough to warrant a change in clinical practice.

Systematic errors may exist in observational studies from the procedure to subject selection, information collection, or confounders. Determining whether a particular bias has actually occurred is usually impossible; therefore, attention is focused on strategies to minimize the likelihood that biases will affect a study's conclusions. The exact level of distortion is generally hard to detect. Assessing whether an observed association is likely to be a cause is based on Hill's criteria, including the temporal relationship, the strength of association, presence of a dose-response relationship, consistency of results across different studies, biological plausibility, etc.

Although consistent evidence comes from the most compelling types of studies (e. g., randomized controlled trial), the reader must evaluate whether the proof can be extrapolated to a specific patient. For other types of studies, even if an association is observed, the magnitude is generally weak. For findings that are controversial across different studies, one possible reason might be limitations of the study design or weak associations.

As with many issues in medical research, the dietary fat-colorectal cancer hypothesis still remains to be answered. Since little harm may be induced from reducing dietary fat intake and other benefits may result, the clinician might reasonably recommend this change in dietary pattern to the patient. Until more definitive information is available, the patient should be notified that the effect of restricting dietary fat on the risk of developing colorectal cancer is slight, since many other risk factors trigger colorectal cancer.

(Wang Hui, Zhang Simin, Jenny Bowman, Wong Li Ping, Zhao Jinshun)

Exercise

Reference

[1]Ahrens W, Pigeot I. Handbook of epidemiology[M]. New York: Springer, 2014.

[2]Carr S, Unwin N, Pless-Mulloli T. An introduction to public health and epidemiology [M]. 2nd ed. Beijing: Open University Press, 2007.

[3]Egger M, Davey G, Altman DG. Systematic reviews in health care: meta-analysis in context[M]. 2nd ed. London: BMJ Books, 2000.

[4]Gordis L. Epidemiology[M]. Philadelphia: Saunders, 2009.

[5] Greenberg R, Daniels S, Flanders W, et al. Medical epidemiology [J]. McGraw-Hill, 2005.

[6]Greger M. The human/animal interface: emergence and resurgence of zoonotic infectious diseases[J]. Crit Rev Microbiol, 2007, 33(4)3: 243-299.

[7]Guyatt G, Rennie D, Meade M, et al. Users' guides to the medical literature: a manual for evidence-based clinical practice[M]. 2nd ed. New York: McGraw-Hill Medical, 2008: 1-860.

[8]Hatsukami D K, Hanson K, Briggs A, et al. Clinical trials methods for evaluation of potential reduced exposure products[J]. Cancer epidemiology and prevention biomarkers, 2009, 18:3143-3195.

[9]Inglis TJJ. Microbiology and infection: a clinical core text for integrated curricula with self-assessment[M]. Singapore: Elservier Pte Lts, 2004.

[10]Jin X, Jones G, Cicuttini F, et al. Effect of vitamin D supplementation on tibial cartilage volume and knee pain among patients with symptomatic knee osteoarthritis: a randomized clinical trial [J]. Journal of the American medical association, 2016, 315:1005-1013.

[11]John M. Last. A dictionary of epidemiology[M]. 4th ed. Oxford: Oxford university press, 2001: 7-8.

[12] Li YP, Li J. Evidence-based medicine [M]. 6th ed. Beijing: Higher Education Press, 2013.

[13]Li YP, Yang KH. Evidence-based medicine[M]. Beijing: People's Medical Publishing House, 2014.

[14]Mahomed O, Asmall S, Freeman M. An integrated chronic disease management model: a diagonal approach to health system strengthening in South Africa[J]. Journal of health care for the poor and underserved, 2014, 25(4):1723-1729.

[15]Maimela E, Alberts M, Bastiaens H, et al. Interventions for improving management of chronic non-communicable diseases in Dikgale, a rural area in Limpopo Province, South

Africa[J]. Bmc health services research, 2018, 18(1):331-340.

[16]McMichael AJ. Environmental and social influences on emerging infectious diseases: past, present and future[J]. Philos Trans R Soc Lond B Biol Sci, 2004, 359(1447): 1049-1058.

[17]Nelson KE, Williams CFM. Infectious disease epidemiology: theory and practice[M]. Sudbury, MA: Jones and Bartlett Publishers, Inc. , 2007.

[18]Rothman K J, Greenland S, & Lash T L. Modern epidemiology[M]. 3rd ed. Philadelphia: Lippincott Williams & Wilkins Publishers, 2008.

[19]Satcher D. Emerging infections: getting ahead of the curve[J]. Emerging infectious diseases, 1995, 1(1):1-6.

[20]Shen H. Epidemiology[M]. Beijing: People's Health Pub. , 2009.

[21]Shen HB. Epidemiology [M]. Bilingual ed. Beijing: People's Medical Publishing House, 2009.

[22]Shen HB, Qi XY. Epidemiology[M]. 8th ed. Beijing: People's Medical Publishing House, 2013.

[23]Shen HB, Zheng ZJ, Zhao YS, et al. Epidemiology[M]. Beijing: People Medicine Publishing House, 2018.

[24]Thorlacius S, Struewing J P, Hartge P, et al. Population-based study of risk of breast cancer in carriers of Brca2 Mutation[J]. The lancet, 1998, 352(9137):1337-1339.

[25] Tibayrenc M. Encyclopedia of infectious diseases [M]. Hoboken: John Wiley & Sons, 2007.

[26]Vicki E, Daha T J, Hans B, et al. Systematic review of studies on compliance with hand hygiene guidelines in hospital care[J]. Infection control & hospital epidemiology, 2010, 31(3):283-294.

[27] Vineis P, Perera F. Molecular epidemiology and biomarkers in etiologic cancer research: the new in light of the old[J]. Cancer epidemiol biomarkers prev, 2007, 16 (10): 1954-1965.

[28]Voloskaya ML. Epidemiology and fundamentals of infectious diseases[M]. Moscow: Mir Publishers, 1990.

[29]Webb P, Bain C. Essential epidemiology: an introduction for students and health Professionals[M]. 2nd ed. Cambridge: Cambridge University Press, 2011.

[30]WHO. WHO guidelines on hand hygiene in health care. 2009.

[31]Wild C P. Environmental exposure measurement in cancer epidemiology [J]. Mutagenesis, 2009, 24(2): 117.

[32]Zhao JS, Ni CH. Preventive medicine, medical statistics and epidemiology[M]. Hangzhou: Zhejiang University Press, 2014.